ASSESSING & MANAGING THE ACUTELY ILL PATIENT

for Nursing Associates

Sara Miller McCune founded SAGE Publishing in 1965 to support the dissemination of usable knowledge and educate a global community. SAGE publishes more than 1000 journals and over 800 new books each year, spanning a wide range of subject areas. Our growing selection of library products includes archives, data, case studies and video. SAGE remains majority owned by our founder and after her lifetime will become owned by a charitable trust that secures the company's continued independence.

Los Angeles | London | New Delhi | Singapore | Washington DC | Melbourne

EDITED BY
CARIONA FLAHERTY
& MARION TAYLOR

ASSESSING & MANAGING THE ACUTELY ILL PATIENT

for Nursing Associates

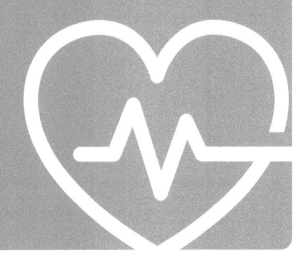

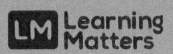

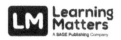

Learning Matters
A SAGE Publishing Company
1 Oliver's Yard
55 City Road
London EC1Y 1SP

SAGE Publications Inc.
2455 Teller Road
Thousand Oaks, California 91320

SAGE Publications India Pvt Ltd
B 1/I 1 Mohan Cooperative Industrial Area
Mathura Road
New Delhi 110 044

SAGE Publications Asia-Pacific Pte Ltd
3 Church Street
#10-04 Samsung Hub
Singapore 049483

Editor: Martha Cunneen
Development editor: Sarah Turpie
Senior project editor: Chris Marke
Project management: River Editorial
Marketing manager: Ruslana Khatagova
Cover design: Wendy Scott
Typeset by: C&M Digitals (P) Ltd, Chennai, India
Printed in the UK

Library of Congress Control Number: 2022945689

British Library Cataloguing in Publication Data

A catalogue record for this book is available from the
British Library

ISBN 978-1-5297-9194-5
ISBN 978-1-5297-9193-8 (pbk)

At SAGE we take sustainability seriously. Most of our products are printed in the UK using responsibly sourced
papers and boards. When we print overseas we ensure sustainable papers are used as measured by the PREPS
grading system. We undertake an annual audit to monitor our sustainability.

Contents

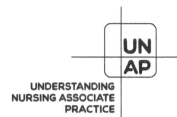

**UNDERSTANDING
NURSING ASSOCIATE
PRACTICE**

Supporting you through your nursing associate training & career

UNDERSTANDING NURSING ASSOCIATE PRACTICE is a series uniquely designed for trainee nursing associates.

Each book in the series is:

- Mapped to the NMC standards of proficiency for nursing associates
- Affordable
- Full of practical activities & case studies
- Focused on clearly explaining theory & its application to practice

Current books in the series include:

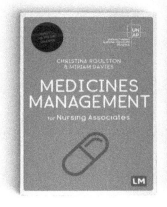
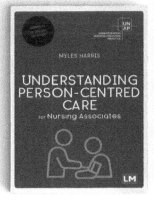
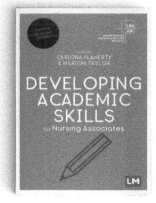

Visit
uk.sagepub.com/UNAP
for more information

About the editors

Cariona Flaherty, RGN, Higher Dip, BSc (Hons), PGCHE, SHEA, is an Associate Professor and Deputy Head of Department at Middlesex University. Cariona is a specialist trained critical care nurse, who has extensive senior clinical and critical care education experience. In addition to her academic role, Cariona is currently a doctoral student at Middlesex University, undertaking research related to critical thinking in undergraduate nurse education.

Marion Taylor, RGN, B.Ed (Hons), M.Ed, SFHEA is an Associate Professor and Director of Programmes at Middlesex University. Marion is a RGN and has a wealth of senior academic experience in leading the development and delivery of nursing and nursing associate programmes. Marion has interest and expertise in supporting students who are also employees, and working in close partnership with employers to ensure students realise their potential.

About the contributors

Lucy Heath, RN, BN (Hons), BMid (Hons), PGCHE, FHEA, is a Lecturer in Adult Nursing. Lucy has extensive knowledge in both clinical and educational settings and is a Cohort leader for several cohorts and Module leader for numerous modules on the nursing associate programme. Lucy has experience in both nursing and midwifery and continues to work clinically in the emergency department and acute assessment unit. Transitioning into education she worked in Practice Education within the NHS for many years, creating accredited modules for nursing staff to assist their development. Lucy is currently a Master's student at Middlesex University, undertaking research related to the use of social media in the nursing associate programme.

Sinead Mehigan, RGN BA (Hons), PGDE, PhD is Head of the Nursing and Midwifery Department at Middlesex University, which delivers programmes for adult, child and veterinary nurses, midwives and nursing associates. With a clinical background in perioperative nursing, she has held positions in clinical practice, clinical education, clinical commissioning, project management and in academia. Academic interests include leadership, anaesthetic and perioperative nursing, preceptorship, workforce development, nursing retention and supporting learners in practice.

Tina Moore is a Senior Lecturer in adult nursing and is the primary and social care lead within the nursing associate programme. Tina has an abundance of experience within nursing education and continues to work clinically. She also has a special interest in clinical skills and has authored a number of books and articles related to nursing skills and practice.

Joshua Sharman, RN, MSc, BSc (Hons), PGCE, FRSPH, FHEA, is a Senior Lecturer at London South Bank University. Josh has worked in critical care, where he continues to work clinically as well as having experience in renal and vascular specialities. Within his educational role, Josh predominantly teaches Biosciences and Pathophysiology. He has research interests in Public Health, focusing on health literacy and the impact of medical misinformation. He has also published articles that explore the use of teaching technology such as AR/VR within the nursing curriculum.

Emmanouil Stafylarakis (known as Manos) is a Lecturer in Adult Nursing at Middlesex University and has an interest in teaching, assessing and supporting students on nursing and nursing associates programmes. His clinical background is in perioperative nursing, specialising in scrub, circulating, leadership and practice education skills in the operating theatres, in both Greece and the UK. Manos' teaching expertise is in the scientific concepts of nursing, perioperative nursing, critical thinking and simulation.

Laura Whitehead, RGN, BSc (Hons) PGCHE, FHEA is a Senior Lecturer and Programme leader for the nursing associate programme. Laura is a specialist-trained critical care nurse with a background in neurology, trauma and cardiovascular surgery. Laura is currently a doctoral student at Middlesex University with a keen interest in the postgraduate education of critical care nurses. Laura is also the creator and host of the *Navigating Nursing* podcast, a careers podcast aimed at inspiring and educating nurses, nursing associates and students from around the world.

Introduction

Who is this book for?

This book is for nursing associate (NA) students, and for those supporting NA students. This includes programme teams in universities, practice education teams, practice assessors and practice supervisors. It is also for registered nursing associates (RNAs) who wish to revise or develop their knowledge of caring for acutely ill adults. It can also be useful for students undertaking a nursing programme, with a placement or interest in acute adult care. Staff supporting learning in relation to acute care will find the case study approach useful, and will be able to utilise the case studies and associated activities within their teaching.

About the book

This book will support the NA student with understanding how to assess and manage the acutely ill patient, with links to pathophysiology, pharmacology and evidence-based practice. It will allow you to develop and enhance your knowledge as a NA student or a NA working with acutely ill adults. This can be useful for NA or nursing students undertaking placements in acute adult areas, or studying this at university. The focus for the book is caring for adult patients with a range of common acute conditions. These are relevant for the NA student or RNA as they can occur in a range of care settings.

Acutely ill adult patients can present in a variety of settings, and caring for such patients is part of the NA role. Understanding how to assess the acutely ill patient, coupled with knowledge relating to the underpinning pathophysiology and pharmacology, is important in order for the NA to safely manage and care for such patients. Pathophysiology and pharmacology teaching forms an integral part of the NA curriculum and assessment, and often students find the application of both to patient care difficult to understand. Therefore, this book will present a series of case studies from a variety of body systems (for example, respiratory, cardiac and neuro) and acute conditions that will look closely at assessment, pathophysiology, pharmacology and nursing management of the patient. This will demonstrate how your understanding of assessment, pathophysiology and pharmacology is essential in order to safely care for the acutely ill adult patient.

Each chapter will present a case study of an adult patient presenting with an acute illness from a range of body systems. This will support NA students with making links between theory and practice.

Each case study will outline how to assess and manage the acutely ill patient within the scope of the NA practice. Links to the underpinning pathophysiology will provide justification for the proposed management and pharmacological interventions for each case study. This will further support the NA student in linking theory to practice but will also provide information on pathophysiology, which often is a complex topic.

The NA role will involve administration of medicines and each chapter will include pharmacology elements. Each chapter will support the NA student to develop the skills and knowledge related to pharmacological interventions when caring for the acutely ill patient.

This book will be evidence-based, drawing from national guidance and best evidence to demonstrate to the NA student the importance of using evidence in support of patient care.

The book will support the NA student with role transition to a qualified NA using a preceptorship approach, and nursing management will address the scope of the NA in the care of acutely ill adults.

Book structure

Chapter 1: Developing your practice as a newly registered nursing associate. This chapter will focus on the role transition from the NA student to the newly qualified NA. A detailed overview of the importance of a recognised preceptorship programme and what it entails will be addressed. This chapter will also discuss the NA scope of practice when caring for acutely ill patients, which will be underpinned by the NMC code.

Chapter 2: Assessment and resuscitation of the acutely ill adult patient. This chapter will discuss how to utilise appropriate evidence-based assessment frameworks and tools to assess the acutely ill adult patient. Frameworks such as the ABCDE assessment and tools such as the NEWS 2 will be critically discussed in relation to their use when assessing and managing an acutely ill adult patient. Adult resuscitation guidelines will be addressed and there will be a discussion on end of life care when resuscitation is not appropriate.

Chapter 3: The acutely ill respiratory patient: asthma. This chapter will present an acute asthmatic patient case study. The underpinning pathophysiology of acute asthma along with links to normal respiratory physiology will be addressed. A comprehensive assessment of the acute asthmatic patient will be discussed, and nursing problems identified. A detailed overview of how to manage the identified nursing problems will be given, with reference to pharmacological interventions within the scope of the NA practice.

Chapter 4: The acutely ill cardiac patient. This chapter will present an acutely ill cardiac patient with an ST-elevation myocardial infarction (STEMI). Normal cardiac physiology and the pathophysiological presentation of a STEMI will be discussed. A detailed overview will be given on how to assess the patient, along with identifying nursing problems. The management of a patient with a STEMI will be addressed with links to pharmacology and evidence-based practice within the scope of the NA role.

Chapter 5: The acutely ill neurological patient: ischemic stroke. This chapter will look at an acutely ill neurological patient presenting with an ischemic stroke. The related pathophysiology will be discussed with links to normal physiology. Assessment and identification of nursing problems for the patient will be detailed. Management of the identified nursing problems utilising evidence-based practice and the use of pharmacology interventions will be discussed.

Chapter 6: The acutely ill endocrine patient: diabetic ketoacidosis. This chapter will discuss an acutely ill endocrine patient presenting with diabetic ketoacidosis (DKA). Normal blood glucose physiology and DKA pathophysiology will be discussed. A detailed assessment of the patient and nursing problems will be highlighted. Management of DKA will be addressed with the use of underpinning evidence-based guidelines and pharmacological interventions within the scope of the NA.

Chapter 7: Upper gastrointestinal bleed. This chapter will present an acutely ill gastro patient with an upper gastrointestinal (GI) bleed. Upper GI bleed pathophysiology and the assessment of the patient will be discussed. Management of the patient presenting nursing problems will be addressed using evidence-based practice and pharmacological interventions.

Chapter 8: Acute kidney injury. This chapter will discuss an acutely ill renal patient presenting with acute kidney injury (AKI). Normal physiology of renal function, and the related pathophysiology of AKI will be discussed. Assessment and management of the AKI patient will include pharmacological interventions and evidence-based practice within the scope of the NA role.

Chapter 9: The acutely ill trauma patient: road traffic accident. This chapter will present an acutely ill trauma patient admitted following a road traffic accident (RTA). The patient will present with a compound fracture and hypovolaemic shock. The related pathophysiology will be addressed alongside completing a primary and secondary survey. Nursing problems will be identified and priorities of care addressed. This patient will lead on to Chapter 9 where the patient will develop post-operative complications following repair of the compound fracture.

Chapter 10: The acutely ill post-operative patient: post-operative complication. This chapter will follow the patient from Chapter 9 who presented following an RTA, who then had surgery for a repair of the compound fracture. Post-operative complications will be addressed with links to pathophysiology. Assessment of the post-operative patient will be discussed and priorities of care identified. Links to evidence-based practice will be made to justify the management of post-operative complications. This chapter will lead on to Chapter 11, where the patient will develop sepsis.

Chapter 11: The acutely ill sepsis patient. This chapter will follow the patient from Chapters 9 and 10, who presented following an RTA. The patient's compound fracture has resulted in the patient now showing signs of sepsis. The pathophysiology of sepsis, assessment and management of the patient will be discussed, utilising evidence-based practice.

Requirements for the NMC Standards of Proficiency for Nursing Associates

The Nursing and Midwifery Council (NMC) has established standards of proficiency to be met by applicants to different parts of the register, and these are the standards it considers necessary for safe and effective practice. This book is structured so that it will help you to understand and meet the proficiencies required for entry to the NMC register as a nursing associate. The relevant proficiencies are presented at the start of each chapter so that you can clearly see which ones the chapter addresses. The proficiencies have been designed to be generic, so apply to all fields of nursing and all care settings. This is because all nursing associates must be able to meet the needs of any person they encounter in their practice, regardless of their stage of life or health challenges, whether these are mental, physical, cognitive or behavioural.

This book includes the latest standards from 2018 onwards, taken from *NMC Standards of Proficiency for Nursing Associates* (NMC, 2018a).

Learning features

Textbooks can be intimidating and learning from reading text is not always easy. However, this series has been designed specifically to help the nursing associate student learn from the books within it. By using a number of learning features throughout the books, they will help you to develop your understanding and ability to apply theory to practice, whilst remaining engaging and breaking the text up into manageable chunks. This book contains activities, case studies, summary boxes, further reading, useful websites and other materials to enable you to participate in your own learning. The book cannot provide all the answers – but instead provides a good outline of the most important information and helps you build a framework for your own learning.

We hope you enjoy this book and good luck with your studies!

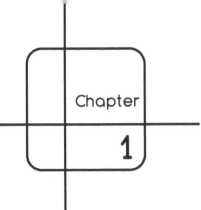

Developing your practice as a newly registered nursing associate

Chapter 1

Marion Taylor and Sinead Mehigan

NMC STANDARDS OF PROFICIENCY FOR NURSING ASSOCIATES

This chapter will address the following platforms and proficiencies:

Platform 1: Being an accountable professional

1.1 understand and act in accordance with the Code: professional standards of practice and behaviour for nurses, midwives and nursing associates, and fulfil all registration requirements

1.5 understand the demands of professional practice and demonstrate how to recognise signs of vulnerability in themselves or their colleagues and the action required to minimise risks to health

1.15 take responsibility for continuous self-reflection, seeking and responding to support and feedback to develop professional knowledge and skills

Platform 4: Working in teams

4.1 demonstrate an awareness of the roles, responsibilities and scope of practice of different members of the nursing and interdisciplinary team, and their own role within it

4.2 demonstrate an ability to support and motivate other members of the care team and interact confidently with them

4.7 support, supervise and act as a role model to nursing associate students, healthcare support workers and those new to care roles, review the quality of the care they provide, promoting reflection and providing constructive feedback

Platform 6: Contributing to integrated care

6.1 understand the roles of the different providers of health and care. Demonstrate the ability to work collaboratively and in partnership with professionals from different agencies in interdisciplinary teams

Introduction

This chapter will consider some of the key concepts that relate to becoming a registered nursing associate (RNA) following your programme of study. It will firstly look at the process of transitioning from one role to another, from being a student nursing associate (NA) to being an RNA, registered with the Nursing and Midwifery Council (NMC). You may have mixed feelings about this transition, and it is useful to reflect on these during this ongoing process.

This will be followed by an exploration of preceptorship, and other support mechanisms available to support you on registration. Preceptorship provides you with a supportive structure as a new RNA, allowing you time and support to adapt to the new role.

Subsequent chapters in this book focus on the role of the NA and student NA in assessing and managing acutely ill adult patients, in a variety of healthcare settings. It is therefore useful within this chapter to look at the scope of practice of the NA, and how this sits alongside the role of the registered nurse (RN), other healthcare professionals and team members.

The chapter will then consider the NA as a practice supervisor (PS) and practice assessor (PA) as defined by the NMC (2018c) and how these roles support nursing and NA students. These might be roles you take on after your preceptorship period, and it is helpful to explore how this change in your role, to supporting other students, impacts on you and your work.

The chapter will finally review the requirements of the NMC for revalidation of registrants, including NAs (NMC 2019). Developing your practice as a NA includes not only developing your NA care skills and knowledge, but also the requirements of being a registrant. Integral to this is the NMC Code (NMC 2018d), which will be explored.

Role transition

There are a number of stages towards the end of a NA programme that need to be achieved successfully before registration with the NMC. These can feel frustratingly slow for some who are desperate to achieve this and work more independently. For others, they feel they are too quick, they feel comfortable as a student and nervous about moving to the next stage. These include:

- passing all academic modules within the programme;
- passing all practice components within the programme including the Practice Assessment Document (PAD) (PLPLG, 2019), required proficiencies and required programme hours;
- awaiting confirmation of these via university processes, often called Assessment or Exam Boards (names vary across institutions);
- awaiting final confirmation of programme completion at an Awards Board (names and exact processes vary across institutions);
- completing a self-declaration of good health and good character;
- NMC registration processes;
- for students who have been funded via the apprenticeship levy, additional processes, currently known as a Gateway Review, that are needed to complete the apprenticeship component of the programme;
- employer processes to secure a post as an RNA.

It is important to keep up to date with each of these processes, ensure you know when each is happening, and what you are required to do in relation to each one. Once all is completed, congratulations! And then what ...? It is helpful to explore how you are feeling and any challenges with this stage within Activity 1.1.

Activity 1.1   Critical thinking

What are the emotions you can identify as you complete your programme and become an RNA and are there particular challenges for you?
An outline answer is provided at the end of the chapter.

It is important not to underestimate the significant transition needed at this stage, and you many have identified a number of emotions and challenges. There are some steps that can help with this process, and support is a key factor which will shortly be explored. Some of the steps that will help you make the transition are similar to those related to the transition you may have made from a healthcare assistant (HCA) or similar, into being a student NA, explored by Taylor (2021a). These include:

- new name badge showing your new role;
- new role showing on the off-duty rota, notice board or similar tools;
- a different uniform if that is local policy.

These small practical steps support you 'feeling different' as an RNA. When accompanied by reflective practice and preceptorship, they should enable and support the change in 'mind-set' that the transition process requires. The important word here is *process*. Whilst some of the key processes do alter things from one day to the next (programme results and NMC registration for example), the transition to feeling and behaving like an RNA is not an instant or a linear one. It may slow at times, halt or even go backwards. This is normal within any transitions, and especially those to NMC registered roles.

The emotions and challenges identified in Activity 1.1 will vary considerably, but it is likely that the majority of new RNAS will identify a feeling of having less 'structure' than when undertaking the programme. As a student NA you will have had deadlines, assessments to work on, reflections to write, placements and university attendance. These will finish as you complete the programme and register. You will have had the support of a practice assessor and a practice supervisor as a personal tutor, university services and a practice education team (or similar). As an RNA these will finish or alter, and different support processes come into place, which will now be explored in the next section, focused on preceptorship.

Preceptorship and support as a nursing associate

In this section, we are going to focus on preceptorship and how this might help you structure your transition to RNA. We will review what preceptorship means, what you can expect, and how to make the most of this experience as you develop your career as an RNA.

The NMC (2020) recognises that the experience a newly registered RNA has in practice, in the period after initial registration, is really important. It can have a huge influence on your journey to becoming a confident RNA. By successfully completing your pre-registration programme, you will have already demonstrated that you have the knowledge, behaviours and skills to gain entry to the NMC professional register as a nursing associate.

Preceptorship is the time after initial registration when your employer provides structured support to help you to consolidate the knowledge you gained as a student NA to everyday practice as an RNA. This will help you develop your confidence and ability to practice safely in line with the NMC Code (2018d). This period of time will be structured with activities that complement and build on initial orientation and induction processes as part of a preceptorship programme. As a newly registered RNA on a preceptorship programme, you take on the role of 'preceptee'. The qualified RNA or RN who supports you takes on the role of 'preceptor'. The activities you will do, during your preceptorship programme, will also prepare you for your future as a reflective, lifelong learner, which is important, if you are to meet requirements for revalidation with the NMC (2019) every three years.

Activity 1.2   Critical thinking

When thinking about your first job as an RNA, what aspects of your role do you think you would need most support with initially? What kinds of areas would be really helpful to cover in a preceptorship programme?

An outline answer is provided at the end of the chapter.

How will I get access to a preceptorship programme?

As you progress towards the final stages of your NA programme, it is worth asking your employer – either an existing one if you are on an apprenticeship programme, or a new employer you are applying to work with – whether they have a preceptorship programme in place for all new RNAs. It is an important question to ask when going for a first job interview. For many employers, being able to offer a preceptorship programme is something they will want to highlight, as it demonstrates to you, as a future employee, that the organisation is committed to supporting your future professional development. You may find that your university will have already flagged some activities in the final stages of your programme, as 'pre-preceptorship activities'.

How is a preceptorship programme structured?

When you start your first role as an RNA, your employer will ensure that you have an induction to the organisation in your first few weeks. This might include a general introduction to the organisation and local orientation to the unit you are working on. Your induction should include a minimum of two weeks of supernumerary practice. Some areas or individuals may need longer supernumerary practice; however, this would be negotiated between the individual, their manager and preceptor. During your induction, you should get an introduction to your preceptorship programme. The programme usually takes between six and 12 months to complete. You will also be allocated a preceptor, who is an experienced nurse or nursing associate, working in your unit, who will support you as you progress.

Over the duration of your programme, you will get protected time to work with your preceptor. During this time, you may work alongside them, both consolidating and further developing your clinical practice skills. You should also meet with your preceptor regularly to spend some time reflecting on practice issues or your practice development. It is important, at the beginning of your preceptorship programme, that you meet with your preceptor to agree on your expectations, and set out a plan for your learning over the duration of the programme. This plan should be tailored to you, and based on the expected outcomes of your programme, and your own learning needs. It is a good idea to agree, early on, dates for interim meetings, where you can meet to reflect on, review and discuss your progress. You will also need to set a date for a final meeting, where your preceptor signs off your learning achievements and relevant competencies.

Alongside working with your preceptor, your organisation may set up other learning activities over the 6–12 months of the programme. This could include study days, focused on enhancing some of your clinical skills. It could also include time for meeting up with your peers – other RNAs, newly qualified nurses, midwives or allied health professionals, to share experiences of working as new registrants. You may also have scheduled sessions with key leaders in the organisation. Many will want to welcome you to your new role, and to share their vision of the organisation, or give advice on, for example, aspects of leadership or future developments. For many newly registered practitioners, the time that senior leaders spend on welcoming them, or sharing wisdom, and the times on the programme spent sharing experiences with peers can be incredibly valuable and stay with you for many years (Odelius et al., 2017).

How do I make the most out of my preceptorship programme?

Think back to your responses to Activity 1.2, where you thought about what you might need the most support for, when you start your role as an RNA. For many new registrants, although you may be excited about the thought of practising as a registrant, you may also feel apprehensive, and question your ability to carry out the many skills that you have already gained in your new role. You may find that you want to focus quite a bit on consolidating your clinical skills. However, it is useful to consider how you develop your professional practice in a wider sense. This is just the start of your career as a registrant, so it is worth developing good habits for your continuing professional development (CPD). There are tools and resources, such as portfolio tools (online or hard copy) that you can use to help you plan your development, and the next sections will look at two of these – one developed through Health Education England and Capital Nurse, and the other based on the requirements for revalidation every three years with the NMC.

The first tool is an online Career Framework tool, developed by Capital Nurse and launched on the Capital Nurse website in 2018. It is free to use for student and registered nurses and NAs (there is a link in the annotated further reading section below). It is designed as a self-assessment tool, which will help you plan, reflect on and record your professional development. It also enables you to get feedback from others, such as your preceptor, peer or service users on nine 'domains' of professional practice. These are:

- teamwork;
- clinical practice;
- communications;
- leadership;
- professionalism and integrity;
- research and evidence;
- safety and quality;
- facilitation and learning;
- development of self and others.

You could use the tool during your preceptorship programme to consider how the activities you are undertaking on your programme help you develop your practice in some of these areas.

An example is presented as a case study below:

Case study: practising communication

In your initial self-assessment, you decide that you do not feel confident in communication skills – particularly where it relates to having difficult conversations. However, you have a session during your preceptorship programme on how to have difficult conversations. During this session, you get the chance to share your experience with other newly qualified RNAs and nurses. Some have had experiences in practice that they are able to share and explore with your group. You then have an experience in practice where you are able to draw on this learning. You get feedback from the person you had a difficult conversation with, on how they felt you dealt with this situation. At your next meeting, you have a discussion with your preceptor on how you feel you have developed your skills in this area. Based on all these learning experiences, you are able to reflect on and get feedback from your preceptor on how these have developed not only your communication skills, but also leadership skills or skills related to professionalism and integrity. You then write a reflection on these learning experiences and upload this onto the Career Framework. When you go back to self-assess your skills, you decide that you have developed your confidence in communication.

This case study is focused on communication, the third of the nine domains within this framework. You can see that there are a number of steps: identification of a learning need, a teaching session sharing experiences, an opportunity to put learning into practice, feedback and reflection with your preceptor. You will be able to use this process for learning within the other domains.

How can I build on the learning in my preceptorship programme?

As you go through your preceptorship programme, think of it as the start of your journey as a registered healthcare professional. You are developing your confidence in applying and building on the learning you have gained during your pre-registration programme. This is also the time to set down good habits in continuing your professional development. As you go through your career, you may well have opportunities to undertake other periods of formal learning, such as modules of study, either with your employer or an education provider. Such formal periods of study should only be the start of your learning. You can increase this investment in your personal development hugely by actively seeking out ways to build on your learning yourself.

For each learning opportunity you get on your preceptorship programme, think about how it helps you build on what you have already learnt before and what you can do to build the learning further after the session. So, for example, you may have had an orientation to the specific medications used in your area of practice. Ask yourself the following questions:

- What do I already know about these medications?
- What further investigation do I need to carry out, to feel confident in managing these medications for my patient group?
- Do I need to spend time with more experienced staff, to talk about their experience of using these medications? Can I shadow a pharmacist for a short time?
- Do I need to access further online information on these medications?
- Can I talk to 'expert patients' about their experience of taking these medications?
- Can I prepare to give patients and their carers information about these medications?
- Could I give a short talk to students – NA students or student nurses – on these medications?

As you go through these activities, it is useful to continually review, reflect on and record how you have increased your knowledge, skills and understanding. The kinds of activities suggested above could be used for so many aspects of your practice.

Going back to the Career Framework tool, you may find that you get learning opportunities in study day sessions, working in your role as an RNA, or working alongside more experienced members of the multidisciplinary team. Some experiences may help you develop your clinical skills. Other experiences, such as those described in the case study above, enable you to develop in a number of areas. For example, you may observe a team leader demonstrating some of the leadership and teambuilding skills you talked about in a recent session with other preceptees. You may also find that you have some powerful learning experiences where something does not go according to plan! In those situations, it is worth discussing with your preceptor what should happen to ensure that things do not go wrong in future.

You will not necessarily be able to think about your learning and development on a daily basis, but it is helpful if you plan, maybe on a weekly basis, what aspects of learning you want to focus on, based on what you are doing on your preceptorship programme – and in practice. As an RNA it can be too easy to focus on the tasks you need to undertake each day, without thinking about how these experiences have helped you develop your practice. It can also be relatively easy to underestimate the degree to which your practice will develop as you progress through the preceptorship programme – and through your career. As you will see in the section on revalidation, this is why it is a good idea to make a record of your learning, and your reflection of the impact this learning has had on your practice, regularly.

Scope of practice

In order to discuss the scope of practice for NAs, it is helpful to remind ourselves of the professional context of the role, which is governed by the NMC. The role is relatively new, identified by Health Education England (HEE), who published their curriculum framework in 2017 (HEE, 2017). The role is designed to bridge the gap in care provision between that provided by unregulated staff such as HCAs and registered nurses (RNs). The need for a role at this level was identified within the Shape of Caring review (HEE, 2015). The NMC became the regulator for the profession in 2017, and published key documents in 2018 related to NA proficiencies (NMC, 2018a), the requirements for NA programmes (NMC, 2018b), support for NA students (NMC, 2018c) and updated their code to bring NAs into line with RNs and midwives (NMC, 2018d). Within the code the NMC identify that NAs are a 'distinct profession' in their own part of the register, but are a part of the nursing team, and exercise professional judgement and are accountable for their work (NMC, 2018d).

The scope of practice for NAs relates to the professional parameters of the role, and the aspects of care included within the standards of proficiencies (NMC, 2018a), and are therefore included within the NA training programme (NMC, 2018b). So to answer the question 'What can NAs do?', the answer is that they can do what they have been trained to do, and assessed as being proficient. Within the standards of proficiencies, employers, RNs and NAs themselves are advised that the proficiencies provide clarity on the NA role, the knowledge and skills they can expect, and how the NA can contribute to care (NMC, 2018a).

It is helpful to consider how the NA role compares to the RN, whose education will have prepared them to meet the requirements of the 'Future Nurse' standards of proficiency (NMC, 2018e). The platforms within each set of standards are compared in Table 1.1 below.

Table 1.1   Comparison of NA and RN roles

Future Nurse: Standards of Proficiency for Registered Nurses (NMC 2018e)	Standards of Proficiency for Nursing Associates (NMC 2018a)
Platform 1 Being an accountable professional	Platform 1 Being an accountable professional
Platform 2 Promoting health and preventing ill health	Platform 2 Promoting health and preventing ill health
Platform 3 **Assessing needs and planning care**	Platform 3 Providing and monitoring care
Platform 4 **Providing and evaluating care**	Platform 4 Working in teams
Platform 5 **Leading and managing nursing care and working in teams**	Platform 5 Improving safety and quality of care
Platform 6 Improving safety and quality of care	Platform 7 Contributing to integrated care
Platform 7 **Coordinating care**	

It can be seen that the platforms within the different professions are similar and complement one another, but it is essential to appreciate the differences in order to understand the scope of practice of the NA. The NMC describe these as 'synergies and differences' (NMC, 2018a).

Key differences are shown in bold in Table 1.1 and include:

- The RN is responsible for *assessing needs and planning care*;
- The RN is responsible for providing and *evaluating care*, the NA is responsible for providing and *monitoring care*;
- The RN is responsible for *leading and managing* nursing care and working in teams, the NA is responsible for *working in teams*;
- The RN is responsible for *coordinating care*, the NA is responsible for *contributing to integrated care*.

Now explore activity 1.3 to have a closer look at the content of the platforms.

Activity 1.3 Interprofessional team working

Select a platform for RN and NAs that relate closely to your area of practice. Aside from the overarching difference in the platforms as above, what are the differences in the exact proficiencies within them?

As this activity is based on your own observation, no outline answer is provided at the end of the chapter.

The NMC (2018d) identify that although the RN and NA play different roles in an aspect of care, they both uphold the standards within the code, within the limits of their competence. This is an important point, that the NA should at all times 'recognise and work within the limits of your competence', as stated within section 13 of the code (NMC 2018d).

It is recognised, however, that the NA proficiencies provide the starting point to the role. Following programme completion and NMC registration, the NA role can be enhanced by further education, training and demonstration of additional knowledge and skills to enhance their competence, as other registered professionals do (NMC, 2018a). This will vary according to the practice setting, and local policies should reflect these additional aspects of care brought into the NA role.

As you use the chapters in this book you will see that the NA student or the NA is working within the interdisciplinary team, and with a RN. The exact nature of the role each person takes in the patient care will vary according to the setting, but will adhere to the principles described here.

To conclude this section, the scope of practice for NAs relates to the proficiencies in which they have been educated and assessed as competent, and any other aspects of care where they have had education, training and are deemed as competent. A further area of practice that NAs can take on to develop their role is to become a practice supervisor and practice assessor, which will now be discussed.

The NA as a practice supervisor and practice assessor

As identified within the scope of practice section, student NAs are supported by practice supervisors (PS) and practice assessors (PA) as identified by the NMC (NMC, 2018c). As an RNA it is satisfying to then support students yourself, and act as their support and role model. The 'Standards for Student Supervision and Assessment (SSSA) identify that all RNs, midwives and RNAs are capable of supervising students, and acting as role models for safe and effective practice (NMC 2018c). This is a valuable role for RNAs, and local policy will determine when this role can be commenced, such as after the defined preceptorship period. The SSSA set out the PS role and how they contribute to assessment decisions. It is helpful to consider becoming a PS, and you can explore your thoughts on this in Activity 1.4.

Activity 1.4 Leadership and management

Imagine you have been asked to be the PS for a year 1 NA student starting in your area next week. What are your thoughts on this? What do you think is important in this role (reflection of your own experiences as a student might be useful here)? How can you prepare to make this a positive start for the NA student?

An outline answer is provided at the end of the chapter.

After some experience as a PS, the RNA can also act as a PA for NA students. This role builds on your experience as a PS, but will require additional preparation for the PA role. It is an important distinction that the RNA can be a PS for both NA and nursing students, but a PA only for NA students (NMC, 2018c). As a PS you will have provided feedback on students to support the PA and assessment decisions, so as a PA you will also use input from the PS. Specific training on the PA role will identify the role and responsibilities in detail, but again it is helpful to explore this yourself, within Activity 1.5 below.

Activity 1.5 Critical thinking

What do you see to be the key differences in the roles of PA and PS? How will your experience as a PS help you when you become a PA?

An outline answer is provided at the end of the chapter.

Acting as a PS or PA is a satisfying part of the NA role, and is likely to provide you with useful material for reflection and feedback on your practice, both useful for your revalidation, which will now be explored.

NMC revalidation

NAs have the same revalidation requirements as other NMC registrants, nurses and midwives. All three professions therefore share the requirements to uphold the Code (NMC, 2018d), and the requirement to keep up to date and revalidate (NMC, 2019). The revalidation requirements are explored by Taylor (2021b) in relation to keeping a portfolio during a NA programme that then links to revalidation requirements for RNAs.

The main components of revalidation are:

- practice hours;
- continuing professional development (CPD);
- five practice-related feedbacks;

- five reflective accounts;
- reflective discussion with your 'confirmer'.

It is useful to review Taylor (2021b) for advice related to organising and developing your portfolio. As an RNA it is useful to maintain this professional portfolio to allow a smooth NMC revalidation when required, which is every three years. This is supported by developing good habits in relation to recording your professional practice and CPD, as discussed in the section on preceptorship and explored within Activity 1.6.

Activity 1.6   Work-based learning

Look at the NMC revalidation website (listed at the end of this chapter), download the required forms for completion, and save these electronically with your name in the document title. Identify what CPD you have undertaken as an RNA, such as a training session, study day, PA training, attending a conference for example. Review if you have received any feedback on your practice, such as feedback from colleagues, other professionals or patients/service users. If you are still a student and not yet registered, this is a useful activity to prepare yourself for registration.

As this activity is based on your own observation, no outline answer is provided at the end of this chapter.

You should develop the habit of collating such 'evidence' as and when it occurs to meet your revalidation requirements. Doing this on a regular basis, and writing reflective pieces after such events, is the best way to meet these requirements. For example, if you have attended a conference, keep the details of this, obtain a certificate of attendance, and then complete a reflective piece on this.

Chapter summary

This chapter has explored some of the key concepts that relate to becoming an RNA, including role transition and how preceptorship can support this process. The scope of practice has been considered, particularly in relation to that of the RN. As an RNA you can begin to support other students as a PS and PA, so those roles have been explored. These can contribute to the revalidation process, also discussed.

This chapter therefore sets the scene for the NA student approaching programme completion, or a newly qualified RNA. The activities within the chapter provide a useful format for personal reflection and review of your knowledge of these concepts. As this book can be used by both RNAs and NA students, particularly those wishing to explore care of the acutely ill adult, this chapter provides these wider issues as a useful starting point.

Activities: brief outline answers

Activity 1.1 Critical thinking

Your answer here will be individual but it is likely emotions may include:

- pride;
- relief;
- happiness;
- worry regarding what next;
- anxiety regarding the RNA role;
- tiredness;
- uncertainty regarding where to work;
- lack of structure;
- loss of your student role, university support and student peers.

Challenges will also be individual but may include:

- securing employment in an area of your choosing;
- wanting a break;
- wanting to go on to further study;
- settling into a new role and a new team.

Activity 1.2 Critical thinking

As with the previous activity, your answers are likely to be individual, but may include:

- Orientation to your new area of employment – both your clinical area and the wider organisation;
- Who is who, within the interdisciplinary team?
- What will others expect of you, in your new role?
- What do I do, in my new role as RNA if something goes wrong in delivering care?
- What will the needs of your patients/service users be?
- What clinical skills will you be using on a regular basis, and do you feel confident in these?
- What are the expectations of you with regard to medicines management?
- Will you be expected to lead care delivery in an area – and a team of other healthcare practitioners and students? If so, how will you organise your/their work? How will you delegate?
- Will you be expected to teach others?
- Will you be able to answer questions that patients/service users and their families might have?
- What is the pattern of work like? Shifts? Asking for leave or days off?

You may find it really helpful if the following areas were covered in a preceptorship programme:

- orientation to the work of an RNA in your employing organisation and area;
- clinical skills consolidation – focusing on the requirements of your particular area;
- medicines management – period of consolidation with your preceptor;
- having difficult conversations;
- leading a team – and delegating to others;
- supporting learners in practice;
- update on health and safety in your organisation.

Activity 1.4 Leadership and management

As with the previous activity, your answers are likely to be individual, but may include:

- thoughts of pride that you have been asked to do this and concerns that you might not be able to support the student as well as others might;
- important aspects of the role you may have identified, including being welcoming and friendly to the student, approachable, working with the student and feeding back to them and their practice assessor;
- preparations for a positive start include knowing the student's name, stage of the programme and what other placement experiences they have had, if any. It is helpful to know how long their placement is for and to be familiar with their PAD. When the student starts, review their PAD and identify any specific skills and learning objectives. It is helpful to have some specific learning opportunities for students in your area of practice identified; these will be in the Student Information Pack or similar document.

Activity 1.5 Critical thinking

The role of the PS is to support the student in the placement, be an effective role model and supervise their practice by working with them. The PS contributes to the student assessment by feeding back on their practice to the PA. The PS can be any registered nurse, midwife or NA, or other registered health and social care professional (NMC 2018c).

The role of the PA is to assess the student and meet with them regularly to record the assessment process within the PAD. This involves some working with the student, and also obtaining and reviewing feedback from the PS and other staff about their progress. You will have had this experience as a PS before becoming a PA, so you will know what type of feedback the PA found useful, and what questions they had asked you. The PA can be an RNA for NA students, or a RN for nursing or NA students (NMC 2018c).

Useful websites

www.hee.nhs.uk/our-work/capitalnurse/workstreams/preceptorship

This website provides a useful guide to preceptorship for those who are about to qualify or are newly qualified as a nursing associate.

www.hee.nhs.uk/our-work/capitalnurse/workstreams/career-framework

This website, which was launched in 2018, will give you access to the Capital Nurse Career Framework. This tool can be used across nursing and nursing associate programmes, and may help you structure your career planning. You can use it as a way of structuring career conversations with your preceptor, or of collecting evidence of your continuing professional development, which will help you as you prepare for revalidation with the NMC every three years.

www.nmc.org.uk/globalassets/sitedocuments/nmc-publications/nmc-principles-for-preceptorship-a5.pdf

www.nmc.org.uk/globalassets/sitedocuments/revalidation/how-to-revalidate-booklet.pdf

Although it may feel very early to start this, it is worth reviewing what you will need to do when you revalidate with the NMC every three years. This website has lots of resources and templates you can use to help you reflect on your practice, professional development and the impact of any learning activities you undertake during each three-year period.

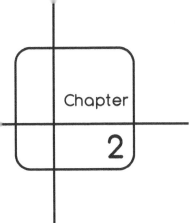

Chapter

2

Assessment and resuscitation of the acutely ill adult patient

Cariona Flaherty

NMC STANDARDS OF PROFICIENCY FOR NURSING ASSOCIATES

This chapter will address the following platforms and proficiencies:

Platform 1: Being an accountable professional

1.13   demonstrate numeracy, literacy, digital and technological skills required to meet the needs of people in their care to ensure safe and effective practice

1.14   demonstrate the ability to keep complete, clear, accurate and timely records

Platform 3: Provide and monitor care

3.6   demonstrate the knowledge, skills and ability to perform a range of nursing procedures and manage devices, to meet people's need for safe, effective and person-centred care

3.7   demonstrate and apply an understanding of how and when to escalate to the appropriate professional for expert help and advice

3.11   demonstrate the ability to recognise when a person's condition had improved or deteriorated by undertaking health monitoring. Interpret, promptly respond, share findings, and escalate as needed

3.14   understand and act in line with any end of life decisions and orders, organ and tissue donations protocols, infection protocols, advanced planning decisions, living wills and lasting power of attorney for health

Platform 4: Working in teams

4.1   demonstrate awareness of the roles, responsibilities and scope of practice of different members of the nursing and interdisciplinary team, and their own role within it

Chapter aims

By the end of this chapter you should be able to:

- discuss the importance of assessment in managing the acutely ill adult patient;
- briefly explain the chain of prevention;
- understand how to undertake an ABCDE assessment;
- identify how to recognise a deteriorating patient using a recognised track and trigger tool, and communication of care;
- outline the guidelines for adult basic life support, and the chain of survival;
- explain the process of ReSPECT when resuscitation is not appropriate.

Introduction

The Resuscitation Council UK (RCUK) (2021a) identified that the average age of patients sustaining an in-hospital cardiac arrest is 70 years, but a quarter (26.7 per cent) are aged 16–64 years; 85 per cent of cardiac arrests happen on wards, in patients admitted for medical reasons (RCUK, 2021a). The annual incidence of in hospital cardiac arrest is 1 to 1.5 per 1000, whereas the incidence of out of hospital cardiac arrest is approximately 55 per 100,000 (RCUK, 2021a). The National Institute of Clinical Excellence (NICE) (2007, page 18) stated that 'patients who are, or become acutely unwell in hospital may receive sub-optimal care. This may be because, their deterioration is not recognised, or because despite indications of clinical deterioration – it is not appreciated, or not acted upon sufficiently rapidly'. The use of track and trigger systems, staff training, and the introduction of a critical care outreach team have been introduced to negate the incidence of patients deteriorating. Tait et al. (2016) identified that assessment and recognition of a deteriorating patient are essential skills for healthcare workers. This chapter will discuss the importance of assessment in managing the acutely ill patient. Identifying how to recognise a deteriorating patient and the role of the ABCDE assessment and track and trigger systems will be addressed. An overview of basic adult resuscitation guidelines will be looked at, and the basics of utilising ReSPECT when resuscitation is not appropriate will be reviewed.

Student tip: Amy

I learnt about the ABCDE assessment while at university, but at the time I did not appreciate its significance when caring for a deteriorating patient. That was until I had a placement in A&E. I was working with my practice assessor (PA) and a patient we were caring for suddenly became unwell. My PA utilised the ABCDE framework to assess and manage the patient's deterioration and used the findings from the ABCDE framework to communicate the escalation of care. I learnt that the ABCDE assessment is a quick, easy to use systematic and evidence-based approach to assessing and responding to the needs of a deteriorating patient.

Chain of prevention

Smith (2010) conceptualised the strategies that support the recognition of, and response to deteriorating patients, which is referred to as the chain of prevention – see Figure 2.1 (Smith, 2010). This five-step approach is used widely across the NHS, and the first stage is education. This chapter provides educative guidance for you as a NA student and you will be provided with further education and training when completing mandatory basic life support training (BLS). This chapter will be following the chain of prevention, by discussing monitoring (vital signs), recognition (ABCDE assessment), call for help (track and trigger). Response will be referenced in each chapter within this book through its application to each chapter's case study.

Let's start by looking at the importance of patient assessment, and monitoring of the six physiological parameters (vital signs).

Chain of prevention

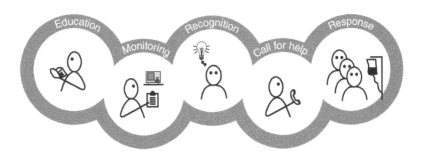

Figure 2.1 Chain of prevention (Smith, 2010)

Patient assessment

The nursing process contains five steps: assessment, diagnosis, planning, implementation and evaluation (ADPIE), in that order (Dougherty and Lister, 2015). The fundamental first step of the nursing process is assessment; without completing a comprehensive assessment, you will not be able to identify and accurately treat an acutely ill patient. Failure to accurately assess acutely ill patients can contribute to sub-optimal care. Sub-optimal care happens when healthcare practitioners fail to accurately assess and understand the significance of clinical findings in relation to the deteriorating patient (Massey, Aitken and Chaboyer, 2008). When a patient becomes acutely ill, this often follows a period of deterioration. In most cases, patients will exhibit obvious deterioration in one or more physiological parameters (vital signs), before the onset of acute illness. Ensuring you consistently complete a comprehensive and accurate patient assessment will help you in identifying patients at risk of deteriorating. There are of course cases where patients collapse spontaneously without any warning, and this is likely related to an acute cardiac or neurological event, such as a myocardial infarct, or stroke. Care of the acutely ill cardiac patient is discussed in Chapter 3, and care of the acutely ill neurological patient is discussed in Chapter 4.

Before moving on to discuss how to recognise a deteriorating patient, **Activity 2.1** asks you to take note of the six physiological signs and what accounts as normal parameters. It is important for you to understand what the six physiological signs (vital signs) and normal parameters are, so that you can appropriately respond and escalate patient care.

Activity 2.1   Critical thinking

Read the following case study, and answer these two questions:

1.   Identify the six physiological parameters (vital signs) which are commonly recorded in clinical practice
2.   Identify the normal parameter for each physiological sign

An outline answer is provided at the end of this chapter.

Case study: Kamal

Kamal is a 59-year-old man, who is works manager of a large consulting firm. He smokes 10–15 cigarettes a day, is overweight and has a history of hypertension, angina and type 2 diabetes. Kamal has been complaining of chest pain radiating down his left arm, and this has become increasingly worse over the last few hours. Kamal's wife calls an ambulance and on arrival the paramedic takes Kamal's vital signs as follows: saturations 92 per cent, respiratory rate 28 breaths per minute (bpm), blood pressure 170/100 millimeters of mercury (mmHg), heart rate 100 beats per minute (bpm), temperature 36.0°C, and Kamal's level of consciousness is alert and orientated.

Recognising the deteriorating patient

Completing Activity 2.1 will ensure that as an NA you can accurately record vital signs, and recognise where vital signs fall outside their normal parameters. Dutton and Finch (2018) highlighted that failure to recognise physiological changes in patients can lead to a delay in the escalation of care, ICU admission and increased hospital stay. Failure to recognise abnormal vital sign parameters are what Loftus and Smith (2018) say can lead to avoidable patient deterioration, and death. An example of this would be a patient dying from an illness that, if picked up early, could have been treated and death avoided. The Office for National Statistics (2022) highlighted that, in 2020, '22.8% of total deaths (all ages) were considered avoidable, that equates to 153,008 deaths out of 672,015'. Although a portion of this number was linked to COVID-19, alcohol- and drug-related disorders, and cancer, the total number does highlight the harsh reality that more work into recognising and responding to the clinical deterioration of patients needs to be addressed. The first approach, as mentioned previously in the nursing process, is assessment, and it is within the assessment that you would undertake the recording and monitoring of vital signs. The RCUK (2021b) has advocated the use of the ABCDE assessment for assessing acutely ill patients. The acronym ABCDE stands for airway, breathing, circulation, disability and exposure (see Figure 2.2). The next section will look at the ABCDE assessment in detail.

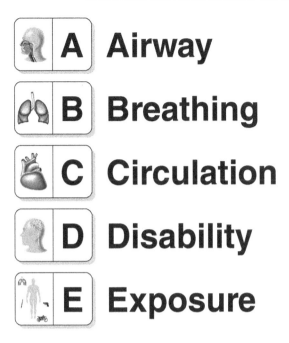

Figure 2.2 ABCDE assessment. Basic emergency care: approach to the acutely ill and injured (Geneva: World Health Organization and the International Committee of the Red Cross 2018. Licence: CC BY-NC-SA 3.0 IGO)

Principles of the ABCDE assessment framework

Smith and Bowden (2017) identified that the ABCDE assessment is a holistic and systematic approach to assessing the deteriorating patient. The overall aim of the ABCDE assessment is to 'identify and stabilise the patient's most life-threatening problems first and instigate further treatment' (Peate and Brent, 2021, page 84). The RCUK (2021b) explained that the approach to all deteriorating patients is the same, and that the underlying principles are:

- use the ABCDE approach to assess the patient;
- complete an initial ABCDE assessment, and then reassess regularly;
- treat life threatening problems first, before moving on to the next part of the ABCDE assessment. For example, if there is a life-threatening problem in part B, treat this before moving on to C;
- know when to call for help, and ensure you call for appropriate help;
- evaluate the effects of treatments;
- utilise all members of the team to ensure simultaneous management of the patient;
- communicate using a recognised and validated communication tool; for example, use situation, background, assessment, recommendation (SBAR). SBAR will be discussed later in this chapter;
- aim, following the initial ABCDE assessment, to stabilise the patient, to allow time for further treatment and diagnosis;

- as it may take a few minutes for treatment to work, allow time before reassessing to evaluate care.

(RCUK, 2021b)

Utilising the above principles provides a holistic approach to caring for an acutely ill patient. The first stage in the above principle is to complete an ABCDE assessment.

Now let's look at how to undertake an ABCDE assessment as outlined by the RCUK (2021b). Please note: throughout this book you will see variations of the ABCDE assessment being used; however, the underlying principles remain the same. As a student NA or qualified NA you must remember to only work within the remit of your role. You must always seek guidance from your PA and/or manager when caring for an acutely ill patient, or if you suspect a patient may be at risk of deteriorating.

ABCDE assessment (adapted from the RCUK, 2021b)

First steps

- ensure safety and adhere to local infection control guidelines;
- ask the patient 'how are you'?
- complete an initial rapid assessment (look, listen and feel approach), this is often referred to as a general and preliminary assessment to address an urgent life-threatening problem;
- seek urgent help if needed;
- if the patient is unconscious, unresponsive and not breathing, call for help and start CPR (if trained) and as per the RCUK (2021) guidelines.

Airway

- look for signs of airway obstruction, paradoxical chest and abdominal chest movement (see-saw respirations), and/or use of accessory muscles;
- central cyanosis (blue colour on tongue or lips is seen as a late sign of airway obstruction);
- partial airway obstruction: air entry is often diminished, and can be noisy;
- complete airway obstruction: there will be no breath sounds;
- *airway obstruction is a medical emergency and you need to seek immediate help.*

Breathing

- look, listen and feel for signs of respiratory distress;
- respiratory distress: sweating, central cyanosis, use of accessory muscles or abdominal breathing;
- measure respiratory rate and oxygen saturation level (per cent);
- assess the depth and pattern of each breath and look for bilateral and equal chest expansion;
- listen to the patient's breath sounds away from the face: chest sounds could include rattling (presence of secretions), stridor or wheeze;
- auscultate the chest – *only if trained to do so. As a student NA you will not be training to do this;*
- look for signs of tracheal deviation. A deviated trachea could indicate a pneumothorax (collapsed lung);
- feel the chest for surgical emphysema (air in the subcutaneous tissue).

Circulation

- look at the colour and temperature of hands and fingers. Blue, pale or mottled could be indicative of a reduction in blood pressure;
- measure capillary refill time (CRT). A normal CRT is <2 seconds, a prolonged CRT could indicate poor peripheral perfusion;
- assess the patient's veins, are they flat and hard to find, or are they visible and full;
- measure pulse rate (HR) and palpate pulses and assess the presences, rate and quality and whether they are regular and equal;
- measure blood pressure;
- auscultate the heart – *only if trained to do so. As a student NA you will not be training to do this*;
- look for external haemorrhages (wound, drains). The doctor will look for internal signs of haemorrhages by using bedside fast scan or requesting a CT;
- ensure patient has access (one or more large bore cannula 14 or 16 gauge);
- take bloods for microbiological investigations and cross match (FBC, U&Es, Creatinine are amongst the most common);
- arterial blood gas (PaO2, PaCO2, Lactate and PH);
- record a 12 lead ECG;
- record urine output (variations of the ABCDE may put this under E);
- record temperature (variations of the ABCDE may put this under E).

Disability

- rapidly assess the patient's conscious level, using either ACVPU (**A**lert, **C**onfusion, responds to **v**erbal stimuli, responds to **p**ain stimuli, or **u**nresponsive) or the GCS (Glasgow Coma Scale). The GCS is discussed in depth in Chapter 4. ACVPU was formally know as AVPU, but C for confusion has been added to link with the NEWS2 discussed later in this chapter;
- examine pupil size – this is separate to ACVPU/GCS. When examining pupil size, you need to look at the size, equality and reaction to light;
- measure blood glucose – this is vitally important when assessing conscious level;
- review any medication the patient may be taking.

Exposure

- assess the patient's skin top to toe and front to back – this will require full body exposure, remember to respect the patient's dignity and potential heat loss.

Additional information

- normally completed after the initial ABCDE assessment, and management of ill-threatening problems;
- take a full patient's history, speak to family and get access to medical notes, use SAMPLE (**s**igns and symptoms, **a**llergies, **m**edications, **p**ast medical history, **l**ast oral intake and **e**vents) to gather information (see Figure 2.3);
- review laboratory results and vital signs.

S	*Signs and symptoms:*	Speak with family/friends/other staff
A	*Allergies:*	May be anaphylaxis
M	*Medications:*	Full list of current medication (dose/time)
P	*Past medical history:*	Obtain notes/GP/Family
L	*Last oral intake:*	Solid and/or liquid
E	*Events:*	Time, onset and severity of illness

Figure 2.3 SAMPLE (adapted from Peate and Brent, 2021)

Activity 2.2 will now ask you to use the above ABCDE information, and complete a full ABCDE assessment on the case study from Activity 2.1. This is an important exercise, and will support your understanding of how to carry out an ABCDE assessment and apply this to a clinical scenario.

Activity 2.2 Reflection

Using the ABCDE approach outlined above, complete a full ABCDE assessment on Kamal. The case study from Activity 2.1. Start with A (airway) and move through the assessment using the systematic approach outlined above and use the observations outlined in Kamal's case study.
An outline answer is provided at the end of this chapter.

Track and trigger

After completing an ABCDE assessment it is vitally important to then know what to do with the information collected and how to escalate care appropriately. In an attempt to improve the recognition and timely escalation of patient care, track and trigger systems were introduced in the UK in 2012. Loftus and Smith (2018, page 77) explained that the track refers to 'detecting an event' and the trigger refers to 'initiating a response'. In other words, track is how you recognise a patient is deteriorating, and trigger is where you escalate care to the appropriate professionals. The National Early Warning Score (NEWS) was introduced as the track and trigger tool in the UK in 2012, and in 2017 this was updated to the NEWS2 by the Royal College of Physicians (RCP) (see Figure 2.4 NEWS2). The NEWS2 has 'received formal endorsement from NHS England, and NHS Improvement to become the early warning system for identifying acutely ill patients' (RCP, 2017).

Physiological parameter	Score						
	3	2	1	0	1	2	3
Respiration rate (per minute)	≤8		9–11	12–20		21–24	≥25
SpO$_2$ Scale 1(%)	≤91	92–93	94–95	≥96			
SpO$_2$ Scale 2(%)	≤83	84–85	86–87	88–92 / ≥93 on air	93–94 on oxygen	95–96 on oxygen	≥97 on oxygen

Physiological parameter	Score						
	3	2	1	0	1	2	3
Air or oxygen?		Oxygen		Air			
Systolic blood pressure (mmHg)	≤90	91–100	101–110	111–219			≥220
Pulse (per minute)	≤40		41–50	51–90	91–110	111–130	≥131
Consciousness				Alert			CVPU
Temperature (ºC)	≤35.0		35.1–36.0	36.1–38.0	38.1–39.0	≥39.1	

Figure 2.4   NEWS2 (RCP, 2017, © Royal College of Physicians, 2018)

The NEWS2 allocates a score to each physiological sign and it is the adding of these scores that leads to triggering an escalation of care (see Figure 2.5 NEWS2 Thresholds and trigger, RCP, 2017).

NEW score	Clinical risk	Response
Aggregate score 0–4	Low	Ward-based response
Red score Score of 3 in any individual parameter	Low–medium	Urgent ward-based response*
Aggregate score 5–6	Medium	Key threshold for urgent response*
Aggregate score 7 or more	High	Urgent or emergency response**

*Response by a clinician or team with competence in the assessment and treatment of acutely ill patients and in recognising when the escalation of care to a critical care team is appropriate.
**The response team must also include staff with critical care skills, including airway management.

Figure 2.5   NEWS2 Thresholds and triggers (RCP, 2017, © Royal College of Physicians, 2017)

Activity 2.3   Critical thinking

Applying the information above, now complete Activity 2.3.
Using the case study from Activity 2.1, calculate Kamal's NEWS2 score, and identify what the trigger of care would be.
An outline answer is provided at the end of the chapter.

Communication of care

Once you have identified a patient at risk, you must now ensure you communicate the needs of that patient, promptly and effectively. NHS (2021c, page 1) defined 'communication as a two-way process of reaching mutual understanding, in which participants not only exchange information but also create and share meaning'. SBAR (situation, background, assessment, recommendation) (see Figure 2.6), was originally developed and used for military communication in the United States, but has since been adopted and utilised as a successful communication tool across healthcare settings. NHS (2021c) suggests that SBAR provides a structured, easy to use approach to communication that facilitates the accurate sharing of information. SBAR has been recognised as a tool that can reduce barriers to communication such as the various levels and knowledge of staff; for instance, as a NA student, using SBAR will support you to effectively communicate with a doctor, or senior member of the nursing team. Activity 2.4 will now give you an opportunity to put the use of SBAR into practice.

S
Situation:
I am (name), (X) nurse on ward (X)
I am calling about (patient X)
I am calling because I am concerned that...
(e.g. BP is low/high, pulse is XX, temperature is XX, Early Warning Score is XX)

B
Background:
Patient (X) was admitted on (XX date) with...
(e.g. MI/chest infection)
They have had (X operation/procedure/investigation)
Patient (X)'s condition has changed in the last (XX mins)
Their last set of obs were (XX)
Patient (X)'s normal condition is...
(e.g. alert/drowsy/confused, pain free)

A
Assessment:
I think the problem is (XXX)
And I have ...
(e.g. given O_2/analgesia, stopped the infusion)
OR
I am not sure what the problem is but patient (X) is deteriorating
OR
I don't know what's wrong but I am really worried

R
Recommendation:
I need you to . . .
Come to see the patient in the next (XX mins)
AND
Is there anything I need to do in the meantime?
(e.g. stop the fluid/repeat the obs)

Ask receiver to repeat key information to ensure understanding

The SBAR tool originated from the US Navy and was adapted for use in healthcare by Dr M Leonard and colleagues from Kaiser Permanente, Colorado, USA

Figure 2.6 SBAR (NHS, 2021c)

Activity 2.4   Critical thinking

Using the information from Activity 2.2 and 2.3, identify how you would communicate care of Kamal using SBAR.

An outline answer is provided at the end of the chapter.

Chain of survival and basic resuscitation guidelines

Having communicated and escalated care for Kamal, let us now consider the chain of survival and basic resuscitation guidelines. The chain of prevention mentioned previously is a systematic approach to recognising, responding and escalating care of a deteriorating/acutely ill patient. The chain of survival (see Figure 2.7) on the other hand is a series of actions to be taken in the event of a cardiac arrest. The first step undertaken is early recognition or call for help; early recognition would include a rapid ABCDE assessment, call and clear communication for help, and the management of life-threatening problems first. Your role as a NA student working under supervision would be to support the recognition of deterioration (completing vital signs) and escalation of care. As a NA student and qualified NA, you will receive basic life support training, and you may at some point be involved in undertaking CPR, either by doing compressions, or carrying out defibrillation if trained to do so. Post resuscitation care would be carried out after return of spontaneous circulation (cardiac output) and when/if the patient has stabilised.

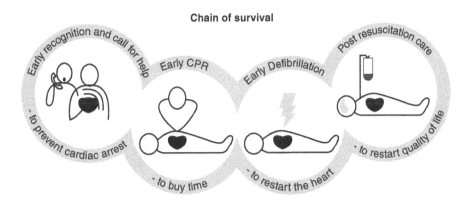

Figure 2.7   Chain of survival (RCUK, 2021c, reproduced with the kind permission of Resuscitation Council UK)

The purpose of this chapter is not to teach you basic CPR, but it is worth drawing your attention to the RCUK (2021d) algorithms for 'adult in-hospital resuscitation' (see Figure 2.8), and 'adult basic life support in community settings' (see Figure 2.9). You will see these algorithms in your local clinical policies and be trained in line with these when undertaking mandatory basic life support training. The RCUK guidelines (2021d) have been updated in light of COVID-19 with this statement 'throughout the pandemic, RCUK resuscitation guidance for *known or suspected* COVID-19 patients has been consistent, advising personal protective equipment for aerosol generating procedures for chest compressions and advanced airway procedures'. For CPR carried out in a non-clinical setting the advice from RCUK (2021d) in relation to COVID-19 is 'if there is a perceived risk of infection, rescuers should place a cloth/towel over the patient's mouth and nose and attempt compression-only CPR and early defibrillation until the ambulance (or advanced care team) arrives'.

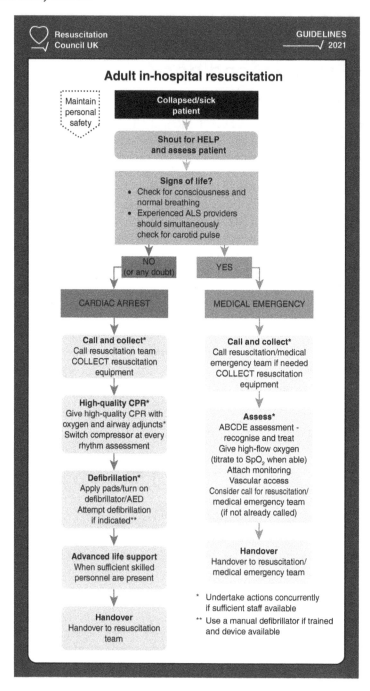

Figure 2.8   Adult in-hospital resuscitation (RCUK, 2021d, reproduced with the kind permission of Resuscitation Council UK)

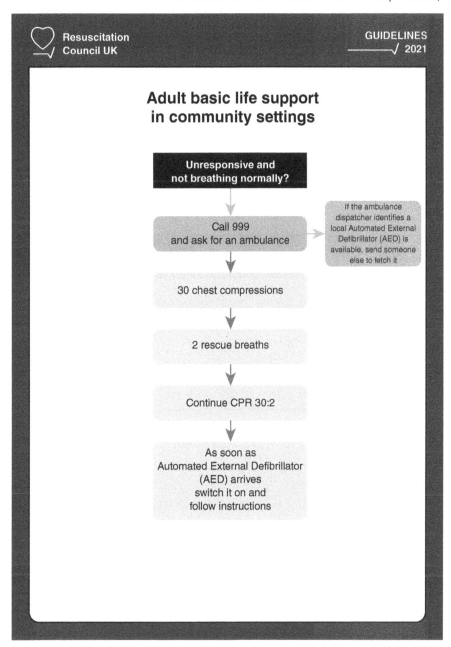

Figure 2.9 Adult basic life support in community settings (RCUK, 2021d, reproduced with the kind permission of Resuscitation Council UK)

Having discussed the chain of prevention, and from briefly looking at the chain of survival, the final section on his chapter will touch on utilising the ReSPECT acronyms to support advanced DNAR decisions.

ReSPECT and DNAR

Cardiopulmonary resuscitation (CPR) was first introduced in the 1960s as a treatment for a person whose heart had stopped, following a myocardial infarction (MI) or similar (RCUK, 2016). However, CPR may not be appropriate for all patients, for example those who are gravely ill, whereby attempts to restart their heart would be futile. RCUK (2016, page 2) stated that 'anticipatory decisions about CPR were recognised as the way to try to ensure that dying people were not subjected to the trauma and indignity of attempted CPR with no realistic prospect of benefit'. All clinical areas, including care home, ambulances and GPs must have a clear policy about CPR decisions. ReSPECT (**r**ecommended **s**ummary **p**lan for **e**mergency **c**are and **t**reatment) is a way of creating personalised recommendations for a person in the event of a cardiac arrest (RCUK, 2021e). This is a process that considers and respects the patient's preferences and the judgement of the clinician. ReSPECT is a multidisciplinary approach to patient care, and decisions are made after several discussions and recommendations. Although the implantation of ReSPECT is not always possible or appropriate in the event of a sudden cardiac arrest, the process could be considered if deterioration and suspected poor clinical outcome is the diagnosis. Making decisions about DNAR should be timely; however, this is not always possible.

Activity 2.5   Reflection

Watch the following video titled 'Joe's ReSPECT Journey – a ReSPECT explainer for healthcare professionals' to learn more about ReSPECT and its application:

https://youtu.be/dp-qOgmBTRw (RCUK, 2021e)

As this activity is based on your own reflective listening, no outline answer is provided at the end of the chapter.

Chapter summary

This chapter began by discussing the chain of prevention and its application to recognising and caring for a deteriorating/acutely ill patient. The importance of understating the six physiological signs and their normal parameters was addressed, alongside identifying why patient assessment is fundamental in reducing sub-optimal care. The ABCDE assessment and its rationale for use was provided, and the use of a validated track and trigger system to escalate patient care was discussed. SBAR as a communication tool was highlighted and this then led to an overview of the chain of survival, including a brief introduction to basic resuscitation guidelines. This chapter was finalised with an overview of the acronym ReSPECT and its use in practice when making advanced DNAR decisions.

Activities: brief outline answers

Activity 2.1 Critical thinking

The six physiological signs are respiratory rate, oxygen saturations, blood pressure, heart rate, temperature and level of consciousness.

Normal parameters are:

- respiratory rate = 12–18 breaths per minute;
- oxygen saturations = >95% (for COPD patients, 88%–92%);
- blood pressure = 120/80 mmHg;
- heart rate = 60–100 beats per minute;
- temperature = 36.1–37.2 °C.

Activity 2.2 Reflection

Airway – clear, Kamal is speaking full sentences

Breathing – saturations 92%, respiratory rate 28 breaths per minute, bi-lateral chest expansion.

Circulation – heart rate 28 beats per minute, BP 170/100 mmHg, temperature 36.0°C, chest pain down left arm

Disability – type 2 diabetic (check BMs), alert and conscious GCS 15/15

Exposure – no wounds identified

Past medical history

Type 2 diabetes, hypertension, angina and smoker

Activity 2.3 Critical thinking

NEWS2 = 7. Aggregated score of 7 or more, indicates a high clinical risk and requires an urgent or emergency response.

Activity 2.4 Critical thinking

Situation:

Hi my name is Amy and I am a nursing associate calling from A&E and I am calling about Kamal who is a 59-year-old man admitted to A&E by ambulance with chest pain. I am calling because I am concerned about his observations as he is scoring a 7 on the NEWS2 score.

Background:

Kamal has been complaining of chest pain radiating down his left arm; this has become increasingly worse over a few hours and his wife called an ambulance. Kamal smokes 10–15 cigarettes a day, is overweight and has a history of hypertension, angina and type 2 diabetes.

Assessment:

Kamal's observations are saturations 92 per cent, respiratory rate 28, BP 170/100, heart rate 100, temperature 36.0°C and he is alert.

Recommendation:

I have started Kamal on high-flow oxygen, completed an ECG and started continuous monitoring of vital signs. I need you to come and see Kamal as a matter of urgency.

Further reading

Steen, C. (2010) Prevention of deterioration in acutely ill patients in hospital. *Nursing Standard*, 24(29): 49–57.

This is a really interesting and easy to read article on how to prevent and respond to a deteriorating acutely ill patient.

Moffat, S., Skinner., J. and Fritz, Z. (2016) Does resuscitation status affect decision making in a deteriorating patient? Results from a randomised control vignette study. *Journal of Evaluation of Clinical Practice*, 22(6): 917–923.

This is worth a read, and provides an interesting insight into DNAR and decision making in patients who are deteriorating.

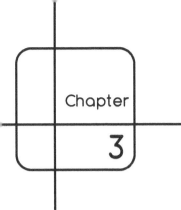

Chapter 3

The acutely ill respiratory patient: asthma

Cariona Flaherty

Introduction

The National Institute for Health and Care Excellence (NICE) (2021) reported that in the UK around 8 million people have been diagnosed with asthma. This accounts for approximately 12 per cent of the population. The Royal College of Physicians (RCP) (2015b, page 2) stated that 'the number of people affected by asthma in the UK is amongst the highest in the world'. In addition, the number of reported deaths related to asthma in the UK remains amongst the highest in Europe (RCP, 2015b). This has resulted in asthma accounting for '2–3% of primary care consultations, 60,000 hospital admissions, and 200,000 bed delays per year in the UK' (NICE, 2021). The increase in prevalence has undoubtedly contributed to the increase in hospital admissions, GP consultations and outpatient clinic services. The British Thoracic Society (BTS) (2019, p.1) highlighted that much of this relates to 'poor management, particularly around the use of preventative medicine'. As a student and qualified nurse you will encounter asthmatic patients across a multitude of clinical environments. Therefore, an understanding of the related pathophysiology, coupled with how to assess and manage a patient with asthma, is essential. The focus of this chapter will be on the acute asthmatic patient. The chapter will start by presenting a case study of a patient admitted to Accident and Emergency (A&E) with an acute exacerbation of asthma, often referred to as an asthma attack. The case study will be central to this chapter and used to discuss basic anatomy and physiology of the respiratory system, and then the pathophysiology of asthma. Utilising the case study, the assessment and management of an asthmatic patient will be discussed, demonstrating application of theory to practice.

Case study: Michael, the acute asthmatic patient

Michael is a 19-year-old student with a long history of asthma, diagnosed as a child. Michael is normally fit and well, his asthma is well controlled with inhalers, and he is currently at university studying history. The past three days Michael has had a head cold, which he was managing with over-the-counter medication. Today Michael has been experiencing difficulty in breathing, with increasing shortness of breath, which has not improved through the use of his inhaler – salbutamol 100 micrograms per dose. Knowing Michael has asthma, his flatmates were concerned and phoned for an ambulance. On arrival to A&E Michael was anxious, dyspnoeic (difficult and laboured

(Continued)

(Continued)

breathing), pale, clammy with the increased work of breathing, experiencing difficulty using his accessory muscles, and unable to complete full sentences. His observations on admission to A&E were:

- heart rate (HR): 120 beats per minute (bpm);
- blood pressure (BP): 100/80 millimetres of mercury (mmHg);
- respiratory rate (RR): >25 breaths per minute (bpm);
- saturations (SpO2): <92%;
- temperature (TEMP): 38.0 °C;
- peak flow: 33–50% of his normal peak flow, which is 600 litres per minute.

Michael was started on high flow oxygen via a non-breather mask, and given 5 milligrams (5mg) of nebulised salbutamol, and 500 micrograms (500mgs) of nebulised ipratropium bromide. Hydrocortisone 100mgs intravenous (IV) and magnesium 2 grams (g) via intravenous infusion were administered. Michael is being treated for severe acute asthma. An arterial blood gas, blood cultures and a chest X-ray were requested to establish/confirm cause.

This case study of Michael will be referred to throughout the chapter when addressing pathophysiology, assessment and management of acute asthma.

Activity 3.1　Evidence-based practice

Defining asthma is complex because asthma can present itself differently across patient groups. Before reading the next section, use the internet and do a search to identify whether there is a gold standard definition for asthma. Consider the following questions:

- Is the source reliable?
- What date was the definition published?
- Do you think Wikipedia has a reliable definition that is used within healthcare?

An outline answer is given at the end of the chapter.

Defining asthma

The Global Initiative for Asthma (GINA, 2019, page 16) suggests that 'asthma is a heterogeneous disease, usually characterized by chronic airway inflammation. It is defined by the history of respiratory symptoms such as wheeze, shortness of breath, chest tightness, and cough that vary over time and in intensity, together with variable expiratory airflow limitation'. The BTS (2019) identified that there is no gold standard definition for asthma, but central to all proposed descriptions of asthma is the presence of more than one of the following symptoms:

- wheeze;
- breathlessness;

- chest tightness;
- cough;
- and, variable airflow obstruction (BTS, 2019, page 2).

Ashelford, Raynsford and Taylor (2019, page 237) identified that at a physiological level asthma has three common characteristics:

- airflow limitation;
- airway hyper-sensitivity;
- inflammation of the bronchi.

Each of these will be looked at further when discussing the pathophysiology of asthma.

Atopic versus non-atopic asthma

Asthma falls under two headings, atopic or non-atopic. Central to each are the presenting symptoms and characteristics outlined above. Atopic asthma normally presents in childhood and occurs as a result of being exposed to an allergen. An exacerbation of atopic asthma could be from exposure to a stimulant such as dust, viruses, pollution, household cleaning products. Non-atopic asthma is not triggered by allergens. Instead, exercise or respiratory infections trigger non-atopic asthma. Atopic asthma is more common than non-atopic asthma.

Activity 3.2   Critical thinking

Look back to the case study and answer the following questions:

1. What type of asthma (atopic or non-atopic) do you think Michael has, and why?
2. What was the cause of Michael's acute exacerbation of asthma?

An outline answer is given at the end of the chapter.

Having looked at the definition for asthma, it is now worth considering the possible risk factors and triggers for asthma. This information is important for you so that when needed you can provide advice to asthmatic patients about ways to minimise recurrent acute exacerbations of asthma.

Risk factors and triggers

Similar to defining asthma, identifying the risk factors and triggers can be complex. Kaufman (2011) suggests that the risk factors and triggers for asthma can be categorised into; host factors, casual factors and trigger factors, each of which is outlined in further detail in Table 3.1.

Table 3.1   Risk factors and triggers for asthma (adapted from Kaufman, 2011, page 50)

Host Factors	• genetic
Casual Factors	• indoor and outdoor allergens
	• smoking
	• respiratory infections (bacterial or viral)
	• parasitic infections
	• lifestyle (diet, weight and use of drugs)
	• occupations (construction workers)
Trigger factors	• stress
	• allergens
	• weather
	• exercise
	• smoke
	• food
	• irritants (cleaning products)
	• pollutants
	• non-steroidal anti-inflammatory drugs (NSAIDs)

Basic anatomy and physiology of the respiratory system

Before you try to understand the pathophysiology related to acute asthma, you must first have a basic understanding of the anatomy and physiology (A&P) of the respiratory system. The NMC (2018a, page 10) states that 'at the point of registration the NA will be able to demonstrate and apply knowledge of body systems and homeostasis, human anatomy and physiology, biology, genomics, pharmacology, social and behavioural science with delivering care'. This section will provide an overview of respiratory A&P, and for further understanding there is an annotated reading list at the end of this chapter.

Structure and function of the respiratory system

The main function of the respiratory system is to inhale oxygen and exhale carbon dioxide. Alongside this the respiratory system is involved in the regulation of pH, production of chemical mediators, production of sound, assisting with smell and protection from external microorganisms (Boore, Cook and Shepherd, 2016). The upper respiratory system consists of the nose, pharynx (nasopharynx, oropharynx, laryngopharynx) and larynx. The lower respiratory system includes the trachea, lungs, bronchial tree and alveoli (see Figure 3.1). A brief description of the function of each of the upper and lower respiratory structures is provided in Table 3.2.

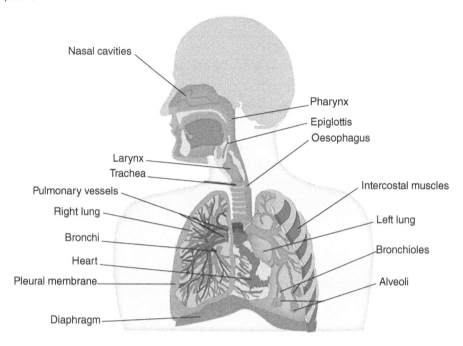

Figure 3.1 Structure of the upper and lower respiratory system (Cook, 2021a)

Table 3.2 Function of the upper and lower respiratory structures

Nose	Provides passage for air entry. Warms and moistens air on entry. Modifies speech and detects airborne odours
Pharynx	Known as the throat. Helps with swallowing, acts as chamber for sound and provides protection for lymphatic organs. Consists of the nasopharynx, oropharynx and laryngopharynx
Larynx	Also known as the voice box. Connects the laryngopharynx and trachea
Trachea	Connects the upper and lower respiratory tracts. Is often referred to as the windpipe and provides a passageway for air
Lungs	The left lung has three lobes and the right lung has three lobes. The main function of the lungs is to facilitate the exchange of gases between the air and blood, and between the blood tissues and cells
Bronchial Tree	To provide a passageway for air coming in and out of the lungs
Alveoli	Facilitate the diffusion of oxygen and carbon dioxide between air and blood

Ventilation

Each of the structures outlined in Table 3.2 plays a fundamental role in the respiratory process, which is often referred to as ventilation. McLafferty et al. (2013) define ventilation as 'the movement of air from the atmosphere into the lungs'. Ventilation has three phases: pulmonary ventilation, external respiration and internal respiration.

According to Boore, Cook and Shepherd (2016, page 269): pulmonary ventilation is the inspiration and expiration of air between the atmosphere and the alveoli. External respiration is the diffusion of oxygen and carbon dioxide between the alveoli and pulmonary capillaries. Oxygen moves into the blood and carbon dioxide moves out. Internal respiration is the diffusion of oxygen and carbon dioxide between the blood and the tissues. During inhalation air flows from an area of high pressure (atmosphere) to an area of lower pressure (alveoli of the lungs). This alternating pressure differences is created by the contraction and relaxation of the respiratory muscles (Tortora and Derrickson, 2017). During normal inhalation (quiet breathing), the diaphragm and external intercostal muscles contract; this results in lung expansion and air moves into the lungs. In contrast, during normal exhalation, the diaphragm and external intercostal muscles relax, the lungs recoil and this results in air moving out of the lungs (Tortora and Derrickson, 2017, page 757). Factors that affect normal pulmonary ventilation are the surface tension of the alveolar fluid, lung compliance and airway resistance.

Surface tension of the alveolar fluid

The alveoli are tiny air sacs in the lungs where gaseous exchange takes place. They are filled with air and lined with fluid, creating a surface tension. Surface tension can result in collapsed alveoli on exhalation, which results in a person not being able to breathe in. Surfactant is a mixture of phospholipids and lipoproteins that is present in the alveoli and its role is to reduce surface area tension. A deficiency in surfactant leads to serious respiratory problems. In premature infants there is often a deficiency in surfactant, leading to a condition known as respiratory distress syndrome (Tortora and Derrickson, 2017; McLafferty et al., 2013).

Lung compliance

Lung compliance relates to how easy it is for the lungs to expand and relax. Surface area and lung elasticity contributes to lung compliance. Lung compliance is effected by pulmonary conditions, as outlined in Table 3.3.

Table 3.3 Pulmonary conditions affecting lung compliance (Tortora and Derrickson, 2017; McLafferty et al., 2013)

Pulmonary Condition	Reason for reducing lung compliance
Emphysema	Destroys elastic fibres in the lung walls
COPD	Causes pulmonary edema
Pulmonary TB	Creates scar tissue
Paralysis	Impedes lung expansion

Airway resistance

The smooth muscle lining of the bronchiole wall plays an important role in airway resistance. On inhalation, the bronchiole wall expands to facilitate the flow of air inwards, decreasing resistance. During exhalation, the bronchiole wall contracts, increasing airway resistance. The autonomic nervous system supports relaxation of the bronchiolar smooth muscle wall (dilation) and the sympathetic nervous system supports contraction (constriction) (Tortora and Derrickson, 2017). The inflammatory mediators released during the onset of asthma increase smooth muscle contraction, which leads to an increase in airway resistance.

Surface tension of the alveolar fluid, lung compliance and airway resistance all contribute to normal pulmonary ventilation. In order to appreciate the need for urgent medical attention, understanding why acute asthma in the main leads to airway resistances is vital.

This section has provided a basic overview of respiratory A&P and ventilation; for further reading on ventilation there is an article referenced in the annotated reading section at the end of this chapter. The next section of this chapter will look at acute asthma categorisations and pathophysiology.

Acute asthma (exacerbation of asthma)

GINA (2019, page 103) define exacerbations of asthma as 'episodes characterized by the progressive increase in symptoms of shortness of breath, wheezing or chest tightness and progressive decrease in lung function, i.e. they represent a change from the patient's usual status that is sufficient to require change in treatment'. British National Formulary (BNF) (2021a) suggests that acute exacerbation of asthma should be categorised to ensure the correct treatment is given. The categories outlined by the BNF (2021a) are as follows:

Moderate acute asthma

- increasing symptoms;
- peak flow > 50–75% best or predicted;
- no features of acute severe asthma.

Severe acute asthma

Any one of the following:

- peak flow 33–50% best or predicted;
- respiratory rate ≥ 25/min;
- heart rate ≥ 110/min;
- inability to complete sentences in one breath.

Life-threatening acute asthma

Any one of the following in a patient with severe asthma:

- peak flow < 33% best or predicted;
- arterial oxygen saturation (SpO_2) < 92%;
- partial arterial pressure of oxygen (PaO_2) < 8 kPa;
- normal partial arterial pressure of carbon dioxide ($PaCO_2$) (4.6–6.0 kPa);
- silent chest;
- cyanosis;
- poor respiratory effort;
- arrhythmia;
- exhaustion;
- altered conscious level;
- hypotension.

Near-fatal acute asthma

- raised $PaCO_2$ and/or the need for mechanical ventilation with raised inflation pressures.

Activity 3.3   Critical thinking

Using the case study of Michael and the categorisation criteria outlined above, can you identify what category Michael's asthma would fall under?

An outline answer is given at the end of the chapter.

Pathophysiology of asthma

Michael's asthma is atopic and therefore the pathophysiology underpinning atopic asthma will be the focus of this section.

The trigger for Michael's exacerbation of asthma was a virus, the common head cold. The pathophysiological response presents itself in phases, as follows:

Bronchial exposure to virus

⇩

Dendritic cell activates T-Help cells to produce interleukins (ILs) IL-5, IL-4, IL-13

⇩

IL-5 activates eosinophils (white blood cells)

⇩

IL-13 stimulate B-lymphocytes to make immunoglobulins E (antibodies) (IgE)

⇩

IL-13 stimulate the production of mucous

⇩

Il-13 stimulate the recruitment of eosinophils to the lung mucosa

⇩

IgE antibodies attach to mast cells resulting in a release of inflammatory mediators

⇩

Released inflammatory mediators are histamine, bradykinins, interleukins, prostaglandins, and leukotrienes

⇩

Causes vasodilation, changes capillary permeability

⇩

Leads to lung mucosal oedema, smooth muscle contraction, bronchospasm, mucous secretion and bronchoconstriction

⇩

Results in narrowing of the airways and obstruction of airflow

Figure 3.2   Pathophysiological response to asthma (adapted from Cook et al., 2019)

The above represents the pathophysiological phases of acute asthma, which normally occur in the first few hours following a patient's exposure to a trigger; in Michael's case the trigger being a virus. During the late phase (normally 4–8 hours after), more eosinophils, neutrophils and lymphocytes are released, which further exacerbates the above inflammatory response. The more exacerbations a patient has, the greater likelihood of scar tissue development and long-term airway damage, resulting in airway remodelling. Asthma is a life-threatening illness, and left untreated it will result in mortality. When a patient presents with suspected acute asthma, it is vital that a comprehensive assessment is carried out in order to identify the priorities of care. With that in mind, using Michael's case study, the next section will utilise the ABCDE framework (RCUK, 2021b). To recap on what the ABCDE assessment framework is, revisit Chapter 2 of this book.

Assessment of the patient with acute asthma

Using the case study at the beginning of the chapter, this section will provide an overview of the ABCDE assessment carried out on Michael.

ABCDE assessment case study for Michael

Airway	• use of accessory muscles
	• difficulty in breathing
	• unable to speak full sentences
	• no visual sign of airway obstruction
Breathing	• respiratory rate (RR): >25 breaths per minute (bpm)
	• saturations (SpO2): <92%
	• dyspnoeic
	• pale, clammy with increased work of breathing
	• using of accessory muscles
	• unable to complete full sentences
	• peak flow: 33–50% of his normal peak flow, which is 600 litres per minute
Circulation	• heart rate (HR): 120 beats per minute (bpm)
	• blood pressure (BP): 100/80 millimetres of mercury (mmHg)
	• temperature (TEMP): 38.0 °C
Disability	• Anxious
Exposure	• No signs of injury or marks to skin

ABCDE assessment discussion

The above assessment is based on the information given in the case study for Michael. One of the biggest mistakes students make when assessing a patient from a case study is that they only use the information that is given and do not mention the other observations/assessments that should be completed. Let us now complete a comprehensive ABCDE assessment of Michael that reflects the RCUK (2021b) framework.

Comprehensive ABCDE assessment of Michael

First steps	• personal safety
	• ask the patient, how are you? If the patient cannot speak full sentences when answering – indicates breathing problems*. **Call for help immediately**
Airway	• look for signs of airway obstruction – the following are signs of airway obstruction:
	• use of accessory muscles
	• difficulty in breathing
	• unable to speak full sentences
	• no visual sign of airway obstruction* *Understanding the pathophysiology at this point will help you understand that exacerbation of asthma leads to lung mucosal oedema, smooth muscle contraction, bronchospasm, mucous secretion and bronchoconstriction – all of which if left untreated can potentially lead to airway obstruction.* **Call for help immediately**
Breathing	• look, listen and feel for signs of airway distress
	• respiratory rate (RR): >25 breaths per minute (bpm) **– this is a sign of airway distress**
	• assess depth of each breath, the pattern, and look for equal chest expansion on both sides
	• note any chest deformity
	• saturations (SpO2): <92% **– this is a sign of airway distress**
	• listen to Michael's breath sounds
	• percuss and auscultate Michael's chest (If trained to do so)
	• dyspnoeic **– this is a sign of airway distress**
	• pale, clammy with increased work of breathing **– this is a sign of airway distress**
	• using of accessory muscles **– this is a sign of airway distress**
	• unable to complete full sentences **– this is a sign of airway distress**
	• peak flow: 33–50% of his normal peak flow, which is 600 litres per minute **– this is a sign of airway distress**
	• trained professional to take arterial blood gas
Circulation	• look at the colour of Michael's hands and fingers
	• assess the temperature of Michael's limbs
	• measure Michael's capillary refill time
	• assess the state of Michael's veins
	• assess Michael's urine output status
	• heart rate (HR): 120 beats per minute (bpm)
	• blood pressure (BP): 100/80 millimetres of mercury (mmHg)
	• temperature (TEMP): 38.0 °C
	• ascertain IV access status
	• monitor Michael's ECG

(Continued)

(Continued)

Disability	• Michael is anxious
	• examine Michael's pupil size
	• complete a rapid AVUP or GCS scoring
	• measure Michael's blood glucose levels
Exposure	• no signs of injury or marks to skin
	• examine Michael's body head to toe for any marks, bruising, wounds or injuries

Activity 3.5   Reflection

Looking at the first and second ABCDE assessments above, compare both assessments and answer the following questions:

1. What would the implications be for Michael if a comprehensive ABCDE assessment was not completed?
2. Why is it important for you to understand the underpinning pathophysiology?

An outline answer is given at the end of the chapter.

Identifying priorities of care for the acute asthmatic patient: Michael

Having completed a comprehensive ABCDE assessment, you will be able to clearly identify the priorities of care for Michael. The priorities of care for Michael, the acute asthmatic patient, are:

1. difficulty in breathing related to severe acute asthma, as evidenced by increased respiratory rate, reduced saturations dyspnoeic, anxious behaviour and increased work of breathing, use of accessory muscles, reduced peak flow and inability to complete full sentences;
2. inadequate gaseous exchange related to severe acute asthma, as evidenced by increased respiratory rate, reduces saturations, dyspnoeic, anxious behaviour and increased work of breathing, use of accessory muscles, reduced peak flow and inability to complete full sentences;
3. pyrexia related to possible respiratory infection following head cold, as evidenced by temperature 38.0 °C.

Reading the above, you will notice that the first and second priority of care are similar and as such, the treatment for both will be interlinked. When assessing and managing acutely ill patients, the goal is to assess, prioritise and treat the main priorities of care.

Identifying priorities of care for the acute asthmatic patient: Michael

Before managing Michael's priorities of care, you need to establish nursing goals. In other words, what outcome do you want to achieve when managing the priorities of care for Michael? The nursing goals for Michael are as follows:

1. Restore normal breathing function/pattern

You will know that this has been achieved when Michael shows signs of normal respiratory rate, equal bilateral expansion of the chest wall, is not using accessory muscles to assist with breathing, is able to speak full sentences and shows normal saturations.

2. Improve gaseous exchange

You will know that this has been achieved when Michael shows signs of normal respiratory rate, normal saturations, improved skin colour and arterial blood gas to measure the partial pressure of oxygen and carbon dioxide in the blood.

3. Reduce temperature to normal parameter

You will know that this has been achieved when Michael shows signs of a temperature within the normal range.

Managing care for the acute asthmatic patient: Michael

Now that you have identified the priorities of care and nursing goals for Michael, let us look at the nursing interventions needed.

Difficulty in breathing and inadequate gaseous exchange

Because both are related to the physiology of breathing, the management for these two priorities of care are interlinked. The BNF (2021a) outlined the treatment for severe acute asthma, such as in Michael's case, as follows:

1. continuous monitoring for physiological parameters: respiratory rate, oxygen saturations, pulse, temperature, blood pressure, consciousness and documentation of these observations and calculation of the NEWS2 score. Revisit Chapter 2 for more information on NEWS2;
2. administering supplementary oxygen to achieve saturations between 94 and 98 per cent;
3. continuous nebulisation for salbutamol (2.5–5mg); the dose and frequency of administration will vary dependant on the doctor's advice and the severity of asthma. Salbutamol is a short-acting selective beta2-adrenergic receptor agonist, and provides rapid relief that normally takes 10–15 minutes to work and peaks performance after 30 minutes. Salbutamol works by relaxing the airway's smooth muscles, resulting in increased airflow. As mentioned previously, the pathophysiology of asthma leads to smooth muscle contraction;
4. if there is a poor response to salbutamol, then add in nebulised ipratropium bromide (500 micrograms); the dose and frequency may vary upon doctors' advice and patient severity. Ipratropium bromide is an anticholinergic short acting drug that produces bronchodilation. The pathophysiology of asthma causes smooth muscle contraction, bronchoconstriction and bronchospasm;
5. intravenous hydrocortisone, normal dose 50mg. Although hydrocortisone can be taken orally, this would not be recommended in Michael's case because he is having difficulty breathing. Hydrocortisone belongs to the group corticosteroids, and works by inhibiting innate inflammatory response; in asthma it works mainly by inhibiting the secretagogue from macrophages, leading to a decrease in mucous production.

The BNF (2021a) highlights that a single dose of magnesium IV and IV aminophylline may be considered in patients with severe acute asthma, but this is only used after senior medical advice.

Reduce temperature to normal parameter

In Michael's case, there is no obvious cause for his pyrexia; however, it can be assumed that his previous history of head colds and subsequent severe acute asthma may be as a result of an infection. The treatment for pyrexia would be as follows:

- as Michael has presented with difficulty in breathing, oral paracetamol would not be recommended. The BNF (2021a) states the guidance for paracetamol is given as follows:
  - for adults (body weight up to 50kg) – 15mg/kg every 4–6 hours;
  - for adults (body weight 50kg and above) – 1g every 4–6 hours.

Additional methods to help reduce pyrexia would be to remove Michael's heavy clothing (with consent) and heavy blankets. Fluids may be considered for patients with prolonged pyrexia to account for insensible fluid loss. Insensible fluid loss is fluid loss that cannot be measured – for example, sweat.

Once the priorities of care are managed and Michael is showing signs of normal respiratory function, it would be safe to then carry on with managing the patient's other problems.

Chapter summary

This chapter started by introducing a case study of a patient, Michael, admitted to A&E with acute severe asthma. The case study was the central feature of this chapter used to demonstrate application of theory to practice. The demographics, associated risk factors, and triggers highlighted asthma as a leading health concern. Defining asthma is complex and is best described by the presentation of symptoms as discussed in this chapter. An overview of respiratory physiology and pathophysiology was addressed to demonstrate the importance of this knowledge when caring for asthmatic patients. The ABCDE assessment of Michael, the asthmatic patient within this chapter, was supported by identifying the priorities of care, associated goals and nursing management using underpinning evidence.

Activities: brief outline answers

Activity 3.1 Evidence-based practice

1. You need to make sure that the journal/book/webpage that you are using is a reliable source; for example, the *Daily Mirror*'s definition of asthma would not be a reliable source; in contrast, the British Thoracic Society 's would be.

2. Guidelines etc. on leading world health concerns such as asthma will always be up to date. It would be unsafe to use a guideline from 2000 when that same guideline had been updated with changes in 2021.

3. No.

Activity 3.2 Critical thinking

1. Michael has atopic asthma, diagnosed as a child.

2. His exacerbation of asthma was secondary to the common cold – a virus.

Activity 3.3 Critical thinking

Michael would fall under the severe acute asthma category, and his presenting signs and symptoms reflect this.

Activity 3.4 Reflection

1. The implications include missed signs and symptoms, incorrect diagnosis, incorrect prioritisation of care and incorrect management.

2. You have to understand the underlining pathophysiology in order to provide safe patient care. For example, if a patient presented to A&E with an MI, and symptoms included shortness of breathing, high respiratory rate, low BP and high heart rate, when looking to prioritise care you would probably assume you would start with breathing. This would be wrong, because the presenting problem is cardiac related, therefore in order to fix the respiratory issues you would need to first fix the cardiac related issues. If you understand the pathophysiology of an MI, you will be able to provide safe and effective care.

Further reading

McLafferty, E., Johnstone, C., Hendry, C. and Farley, A. (2013) Respiratory system part 1: pulmonary ventilation. *Nursing Standard*, 27(22): 40–47

This article covers A&P of the respiratory system and the mechanics of ventilation in more depth.

McLafferty, E., Johnstone, C., Hendry, C. and Farley, A. (2013) Respiratory system part 2: gaseous exchange. *Nursing Standard*, 27(23): 35–42.

This article provides an excellent overview of gaseous exchange, transport of oxygen and carbon dioxide and internal and external respiration.

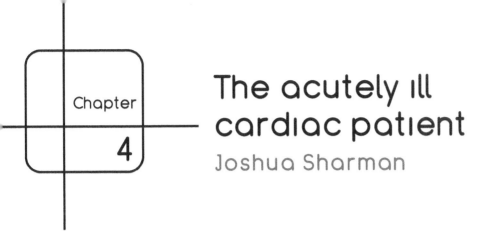

Chapter 4

The acutely ill cardiac patient

Joshua Sharman

NMC STANDARDS OF PROFICIENCY FOR NURSING ASSOCIATES

This chapter will address the following platforms and proficiencies:

Platform 2: Promoting health and preventing ill health

2.2   promote preventative health behaviours and provide information to support people in making informed choices to improve their mental, physical and behavioural health and well-being

Platform 3: Provide and monitor care

3.2   demonstrate and apply knowledge of body systems and homeostasis, human anatomy and physiology, biology, genomics, pharmacology, social and behavioural sciences when delivering care

3.3   recognise and apply knowledge of commonly encountered mental, physical, behavioural and cognitive health conditions when delivering care

3.4   demonstrate the knowledge, communication and relationship management skills required to provide people, families and carers with accurate information that meets their needs before, during and after a range of interventions.

3.7   demonstrate and apply an understanding of how and when to escalate the appropriate professional for expert help and advice

3.11   demonstrate the ability to recognise when a person's condition has improved or deteriorated by undertaking health monitoring. Interpret, promptly respond, share findings and escalate if needed

Chapter aims

After reading this chapter you will be able to:

- understand the anatomy and physiology of the cardiac system;
- understand the pathophysiology of coronary heart disease, particularly ST elevation myocardial infarction (STEMI);
- have an awareness of ECG interpretation in relation to STEMI;
- demonstrate your ability to contribute to an assessment of the cardiac patient;
- identify the priorities of care to treat a patient with STEMI and the role of the nursing associate within this.

Introduction

This chapter will outline the prevalence of cardiovascular diseases in the UK and identify those who are at a higher risk. Cardiac anatomy, physiology and pathophysiology will be discussed with specific focus on myocardial infarction (heart attack). A case study is presented, giving you the opportunity to critically think about the assessment and management of a patient presenting with a ST elevation myocardial infarction (STEMI). There are a number of other acute cardiac conditions which cannot be included within the limitations of this chapter, but it is hoped that the principles of assessment and management covered can be applied to other conditions. This chapter will be useful for nursing associate (NA) students undergoing a placement within cardiology or caring for acute cardiac patients, or a registered nursing associate (RNA) wishing to develop their practice in this area.

Coronary heart disease (CHD) is one of the UK's leading causes of death and the most common cause of premature death, with 1 in 8 men and 1 in 15 women dying from CHD each year, killing more women than breast cancer. CHD is responsible for 64,000 deaths each year; on average that's 175 people each day, or around one death every eight minutes. CHD death rates are highest within the north of England and Scotland (British Heart Foundation, 2021).

CHD is an umbrella term that covers three medical conditions: angina (stable & unstable) and myocardial infarction (heart attack). Myocardial infarctions (MI) result in 100,000 hospital admissions each year in the UK, averaging 280 admissions each day, around one every five minutes (British Heart Foundation, 2021).

There are many risk factors that increase an individual's likelihood of developing CHD such as high blood pressure (hypertension), diabetes, high cholesterol, air pollution, smoking, overweight/obesity, poor diet and lack of exercise, along with impaired renal function, old age, gender, family history and ethnicity.

The NHS Long Term Plan (2019) outlines how cardiovascular disease (CVD) is the single biggest area where the NHS can save lives over the next ten years. Health Education England also aims to improve the diagnosis of heart failure and heart valve diseases by supporting the earlier detection of heart failure through recognition and assessment of the disease

(Health Education England, 2021). As a nursing associate (NA), part of your role is to record and interpret vital signs and undertake ECG recording, recognise emergency situations and understand when to escalate to appropriate professional help and advice (Nursing and Midwifery Council, 2018a).

As you will learn throughout this chapter, a STEMI is the medical term for a type of heart attack or myocardial infarction (MI). The incidence of STEMI has been declining over the past 20 years and in-hospital mortality has declined from around 20 per cent to nearer 5 per cent; this has been because of several factors such as improved drug therapy and speed of access to better treatments (NICE, 2014).

In order to explore the assessment and management of a patient with STEMI, we will first focus on a patient case study, Mrs Patel.

Case study: Mrs Patel, the acutely ill cardiac patient

A 62-year-old female has been admitted onto a cardiac ward for investigation of chest pain over the past three days. The patient has reported a seven-day history of increasing fatigue on exertion and shortness of breath; she describes that going to the toilet has become very difficult. The patient is a type-II diabetic, her condition controlled with insulin, and has peripheral vascular disease.

Mrs Patel is of South Indian heritage and is categorised as obese when using a body mass index. She reports that within the last six months her diabetes has been uncontrolled, and her blood sugar is often between 15 and 20 in the evenings. She takes very little exercise and relies on her son and daughter to support her with her activities of daily living, such as personal care, eating and drinking and the administration of her medication.

Mrs Patel has awoken this morning and has complained of increasing chest pain; you immediately notice that she is clammy. The RN that you are working with requests that you complete a set of observations and carry out an ECG.

Mrs Patel's observations are as follows:

respiratory rate: 23;
oxygen saturation: 96% (scale 1);
oxygen: room air;
blood pressure: 160/96;
pulse: 106;
consciousness: alert;
temperature: 36.2°C.

The RN gives you an ECG that was performed yesterday. They ask that you give this, along with the ECG obtained today, to the medical team to compare. The RN also requests that you explain that the patient is complaining of worsening chest pain and ask that Mrs Patel is reviewed urgently.

The two ECGs are displayed in Figures 4.1 and 4.2. These are reviewed by the medical team, who then report that there are changes, and that ST-elevation is observable on the most recent ECG, confirming a STEMI.

(Continued)

(Continued)

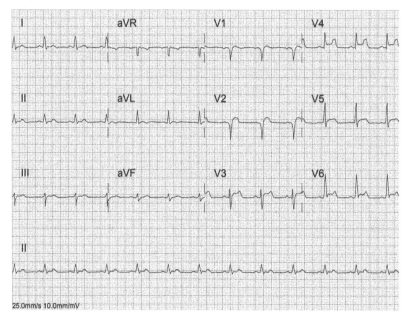

Figure 4.1   ECG showing a ST elevation (antero-lateral MI) (this is a simulated image, used with permission from Laerdal Medical, 2011)

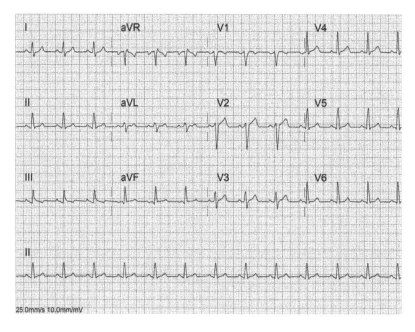

Figure 4.2   ECG taken on admission three days ago – normal ECG (this is a simulated image, used with permission from Laerdal Medical, 2011)

Before we go on to the relevant anatomy, it is helpful to explore your current knowledge, and review the information in the above case study by completing Activity 4.1.

Activity 4.1 Critical thinking

- Are Mrs Patel's observations normal?
- What are your immediate concerns?

An outline answer is given at the end of the chapter.

Before you move on to the next section in the chapter, take some time to think about the risk factors that were identified within the introduction and how these may apply to the case study above.

Cardiac anatomy and physiology

To assess and care for Mrs Patel, an understanding of cardiac anatomy is essential. This is important for patients presenting in an emergency with STEMI, as invasive interventions can be delivered very quickly, and patients and their relatives will require support to understand what a STEMI is and how it is treated, along with the severity of the condition.

The heart is about the size of your fist and is located on the left side of your chest (thorax), towards the front (anterior) of your lungs. The heart is rotated at about 30 degrees, meaning that the heart is slightly twisted. Most of the heart is made up of muscle, specifically 'cardiac muscle', and this muscular pump is required to pump blood around the body.

The heart is split into four chambers, each pumping blood to a different location; for example, the right atrium pumps blood to the right ventricle, the right ventricle then pumps blood to the lungs via the pulmonary artery. A similar process happens on the left side of the heart.

The four chambers are:

- right atrium (RA);
- left atrium (LA);
- right ventricle (RV);
- left ventricle (LV).

It is helpful to be clear where each of the four chambers is located and the different blood vessels that bring blood into the heart (veins), take it away (arteries) and the blood supply to the heart itself. This is shown in Figure 4.3.

Due to the rotation of the heart, the RV is the structure that is the closest to the chest wall. The RA and LA, the two chambers located at the top of the heart, are smaller, pushing blood into the larger chambers, RV and LV, which are located at the bottom of the heart and push blood away from the heart, either to your lungs or the rest of your body.

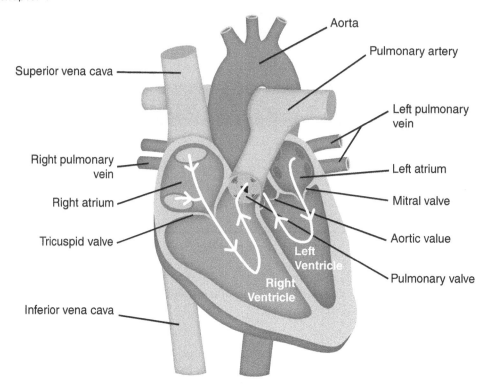

Figure 4.3   Anatomy of the heart (Cook, 2021a)

Figure 4.4 shows how blood passes through the heart. Deoxygenated blood enters via the inferior and superior vena cava into the right atrium; following contraction of the upper chambers blood is pushed in the right ventricle. The blood then flows via the pulmonary artery and becomes oxygenated in the lungs before re-entering the left side of the heart by the pulmonary vein. Once blood is in the left atrium, there is another contraction of the upper two chambers, which subsequently pushes blood into the left ventricle, and once in the left ventricle the ventricles contract and this pushes blood out of the heart to the body.

Like all organs, the heart requires a constant flow of blood to maintain the ability to function. The heart receives blood flow from vessels called the coronary arteries; there are two main coronary arteries called the left and right coronary artery, these are shown in Figure 4.5. The left coronary artery runs down the left side of the heart, and the right coronary artery runs down the right side of the heart.

Blood flows from the coronary arteries and passes through the cardiac capillary bed and then back to the cardiac veins; this deoxygenated blood then drains into the right atrium. Once blood is within the cardiac capillary bed, the thin membranes of the capillaries allow for diffusion of oxygen and carbon dioxide as well as electrolytes and glucose, to supply the cardiac muscle.

If blood flow is interrupted to an area of cardiac muscle, a blocked blood vessel for example, that area will start to die (infarction) and result in that part of the heart pumping ineffectively.

Pulmonary artery

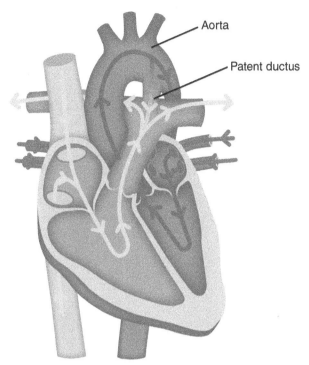

Figure 4.4 Blood flow through the heart (Cook, 2021a)

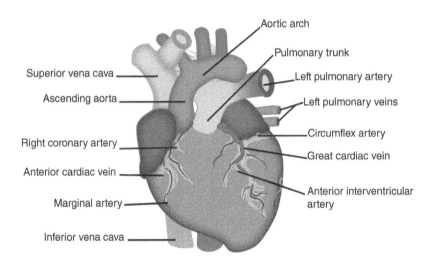

Figure 4.5 The coronary vessels (Cook, 2021a)

Electrical conduction

The heart relies on electrical stimulus to beat; these electrical signals essentially cause cardiac muscle to contract, resulting in a heartbeat and therefore movement of blood around the body.

These electrical impulses start at 'nodes' and travel along nerves; as one cell starts to contract, the neighbouring cells around it will do the same and this results in what is called depolarisation (contraction) of the heart (see Figure 4.6).

This process starts with the sino-atrial (SA) node, located in the upper right corner of the right atrium. This node is known as the 'pacemaker' and naturally generates an electrical impulse of 60–100 times per minute. This initial electrical impulse travels from the SA node to the neighbouring cells, the cells depolarise, which results in contraction of the atrial heart muscle. This initial impulse, however, only travels to the atria; there is a short pause before the impulse then continues along the ventricles. This short pause enables blood to travel from the atria to the ventricles; essentially the ventricles take a short period of time to fill with blood. This is where another node called the atrioventricular (AV) node has a role. The AV node is responsible for pausing the electrical impulse before sending it to the ventricles, essentially stopping them from beating too quickly. The AV node is located just below the right atrium. Following the pause of the impulse by the AV node, the impulse progesses down the bundle of His and along the purkinje fibres, which results in depolarisation, resulting in ventricular depolarisation and contraction of the ventricles, which then pump blood to the lungs and around the body.

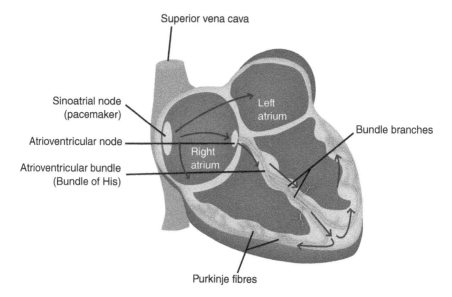

Figure 4.6   Electrical conduction pathway within the heart (Cook, 2021a)

Now we have reviewed normal anatomy and physiology, we will move on to cardiac pathophysiology.

Before you move on to the pathophysiology, where we will begin to look at the disease processes, take some time to explore the further reading identified in this chapter; this will help you further consolidate your learning on the anatomy of the cardiovascular system.

Pathophysiology

Atherosclerosis

Most CHD is due to a condition called atherosclerosis. Atherosclerosis is a complex condition which affects the arteries of the heart but can also cause cerebrovascular diseases (diseases of the vessels in the brain). The condition causes the build-up of cholesterol on the inside of the artery wall. This build-up ultimately results in a narrowing of the blood vessel supplying the heart with blood and therefore reduces blood flow to heart muscle.

The cholesterol results in plaque 'atheroma', which usually evolves over several years; inflammation arises within the artery wall because of damage caused by plaque and blood flow is affected.

Figure 4.7 shows the building up of plaque on the inside of an artery wall that causes narrowing of the vessel, effecting blood flow through the artery. Part A of the image shows normal blood flow through an artery, Part B shows the build-up of artheroma, which limits the blood flow through the vessel. When this happens to the coronary blood vessels within the heart, the reduction in blood flow results in strain on the heart muscle. The strain essentially starts to result in heart muscle not working as effectively and in some cases part of the heart muscle can start to infarct, as has occurred for Mrs Patel.

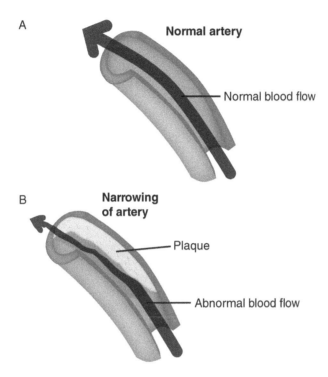

Figure 4.7   Atheroma within an artery (Cook, 2021a)

Ischaemia/Infarction

When we talk about death to heart tissue, this is usually because of a blockage within one of the coronary arteries; this blockage means that the heart muscle is becoming starved of oxygen and this lack of oxygen results in death to the tissue.

There are many different terms used to describe death to heart tissue:

- *Ischaemia* is the inadequate blood supply to a certain part of the body, and this would usually result in tissue dying if blood flow is not restored. This can be within the heart or other parts of the body such as the brain (stroke) and a limb (critical limb ischemia).
- Another term you may hear to describe the death of tissue is *infarction*, which is similar to ischemia; however, if there is an infarction this implies that there is an obstruction within a blood vessel which is supplying an organ and this blockage is usually a thrombus or embolus as a result of atherosclerosis. An infarction would typically mean that the blockage within the blood vessels is causing the organ tissue to die because of a lack of oxygen.

This is shown in Figure 4.8, where a coronary artery has become partly or fully occluded because of atherosclerosis. The image on the left identifies the area where the vessel has been occluded and therefore the potential damage that can be done to the heart tissue.

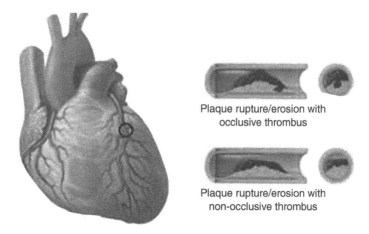

Plaque rupture/erosion with
occlusive thrombus

Plaque rupture/erosion with
non-occlusive thrombus

Figure 4.8　Atherosclerosis within the coronary vessels (Thygesen et al., 2018)

Before moving on to further pathophysiology it is helpful to review your learning so far and your knowledge of the risk factors in relation to cardiac disease, and relate this to Mrs Patel in the following activity.

Activity 4.2　Evidence-based practice and research

Refer back to the case study at the beginning of the chapter, and make your own notes on what risk factors for cardiac disease can be identified for Mrs Patel.

An outline answer is given at the end of the chapter.

Acute coronary syndromes

Acute coronary syndrome (ACS) is a term used to describe a range of conditions that are associated with a reduction in blood supply to the heart. ACS is subdivided into categories, depending on the clinical presentation of a patient, and would depend on ECG findings and biomarkers such as blood tests. Figure 4.9 demonstrates the different types of ECG changes that patients can present with; this knowledge is used to determine the diagnosis and therefore treatment.

ACS includes a range of conditions such as unstable angina and myocardial infarction (MI), of which there are two types: non ST elevation myocardial infarction (NSTEMI) and ST elevation myocardial infarction (STEMI). The broader term of coronary heart disease (CHD) includes all the above as well as stable angina; however, stable angina is not seen to be an acute cardiac episode that requires immediate intervention.

The management of patients with ACS has improved over the last few decades as the knowledge and understanding of the physiology process has developed. As mentioned above, ACS is split into three different subcategories, which are outlined below:

- ST elevation MI (STEMI) – patients who are experiencing a STEMI are experiencing an acute myocardial ischemia. It suggests that there is cardiac ischemia. It is diagnosed with ST elevation found on an ECG, coupled with the release of biomarkers found in blood tests, following part of the heart muscle starting to infarct;
- non-ST elevation MI (NSTEMI) – patients suffering an NSTEMI are also experiencing acute myocardial ischemia; however, there is no ST elevation recorded on an ECG, but this could however present as ECG abnormalities such as T wave inversion or ST depression, as shown in Figure 4.9. There is also the release of biomarkers found following cardiac infarction;
- unstable angina – patients experiencing unstable angina are also experiencing acute myocardial ischemia. This would usually present with ECG changes, usually determined by previous ECGs; however, there is no ST elevation (but typically present with ST depression or T wave inversion). There is also no release of biomarkers found following cardiac infarction.

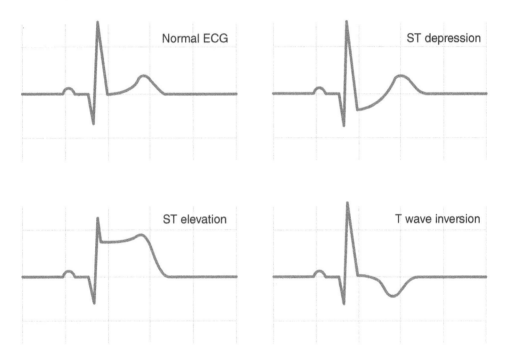

Figure 4.9 ECG changes related to ACS (Cook, 2021b)

ST elevation presentation

The presentation of a STEMI in patients can vary from person to person; sometimes the symptoms can develop over a couple of days and in other cases it can be a very sudden onset. Typically, patients would present with chest pain, as has Mrs Patel. The pain can be crushing and possibly the pain is radiating down the arm, jaw or back. Other symptoms may be malaise and fatigue as well as shortness of breath. It is important to remember that certain patients may present atypically; for example, diabetics may not have chest pain and describe an uncomfortable feeling in their chest, whilst some patients may also have nausea and vomiting.

Assessment of the acutely ill cardiac patient

A STEMI is a serious medical emergency, and it is essential that as an NA or NA student you can recognise the pathophysiological changes and have an understanding of how these are assessed. The development of the skills required to assess a cardiac patient are essential in ensuring subsequent management of these patients, and this requires knowledge of normal anatomy, and pathophysiology as covered in this chapter. Effective assessment is vital and we will now explore the components of a cardiac assessment of Mrs Patel:

- ECG;
- ABCDE assessment;
- pain assessment.

Electrocardiogram (ECG) recognition

An ECG is a visual representation of the electrical conduction occurring over one cardiac cycle, explained earlier, specifically the conduction of electrical impulses from the artia to the ventricles. An ECG is made up of five waveforms, which are labelled P, Q, R, S and T; the middle letters Q, R, S are usually referred to as a complex – the QRS complex.

The P wave represents the contraction of the upper two chambers (atria), the QRS complex represents contraction of the bottom two chambers (the ventricles) and a T wave represents the recharging or repolarisation (recovery) of the heart cells as shown in Figure 4.10.

The five different wave forms together represent one heartbeat. It is important to remember that an ECG trace is only showing you the travel of electrical activity through the cardiac conduction system – it isn't showing you the mechanical contraction of the heart that follows electrical conduction. For example, you could have a 'relatively' normal ECG without mechanical contraction as the heart could be ineffective at mechanically pumping blood around the body; therefore it is important that a full and complete assessment is carried out on all patients who present with potential cardiac conditions.

The ABCDE approach

When assessing Mrs Patel, an 'ABCDE' approach should be used. This requires you to ask yourself questions and, if abnormal findings are found within the assessment, interventions may be necessary (RCUK, 2021b). While completing an ABCDE assessment, it is important to recognise when expert help is required, and this should always be sought as soon as possible. As an NA or NA student, the ABCDE assessment should be completed under the direct supervision of a registered nurse (RN). The ABCDE approach is now explained.

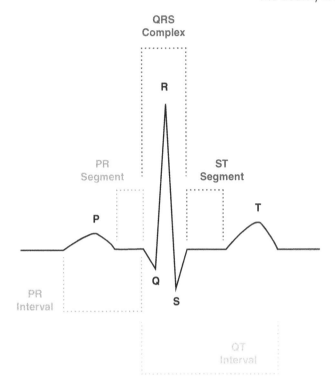

Figure 4.10 PQRS complex (Wettstein, 2020, CC BY-NC-ND 4.0)

- **A**irway: is the airway patent (open)? Is the patient able to maintain their own airway?
- **B**reathing: is the patient breathing? If so, what is the respiratory rate and oxygen saturation? Also note the depth and symmetry of chest expansion;
- **C**irculation: assess the pulse rate, rhythm and volume, blood pressure, capillary refill time, urine output; if required attach the patient to a cardiac monitor and perform a 12-lead ECG;
- **D**isability: establish the patient's level of consciousness using alert, confusion, voice, pain, unresponsive;
- **E**xposure: record the temperature, full head to toe assessment and exposure of the body to ensure no other injuries are present.

It is important that you can recognise when to call for help. The aim of an ABCDE assessment is that you access a patient in order of priority and attempt to intervene when required. It is also important to understand that a fundamental component of providing care is to recognise when you need specialist help or when you feel you are practising outside of your competence. Depending on the situation, you may need assistance from the medical emergency team, critical care outreach team or a senior healthcare professional. If you are practising within the community, you will need to rely on the ambulance service for emergency care by calling '999'.

Pain assessment

When assessing Mrs Patel for pain there are several factors that need to be considered. When patients present with a form of chest pain, understanding the pain can be critical in determining stable and unstable cardiac conditions, and ruling out possible non-cardiac conditions. Pain can be difficult to measure as it is subjective: one person's pain can be different from another's; however, to develop a full understanding of an individual's pain, a pain assessment tool should be used. The PQRST method is a valuable tool in understanding a patient's pain, allowing them to describe the type of pain they are feeling (Barrett, Gretton and Quinn, 2006). The PQRST method is:

Provocation/Palliation
What were you doing when the pain started? What caused it? What makes it better or worse? What seems to trigger it?
Quality/Quantity
What does it feel like? Is it a sharp, dull, stabbing, burning, crushing etc. type of pain?
Region/Radiation
Where is the pain located? Does it radiate anyway? Does it move around? Did it start somewhere else?
Severity scale
How severe is the pain on a scale of 1–10? How bad was it at its worst? How long does it last for?
Timing
When/at what time did the pain start? Have you experienced anything like this before? When does it occur? Before or after meals?

Having assessed Mrs Patel, she is then referred to the critical care outreach team using a situation background assessment recommendation (SBAR) handover (Institute for Innovation & Improvement, 2017). SBAR is an easy to use, structured communication tool that allows for information to be communicated accurately between individuals. There are prompts within four sections to ensure that you are sharing concise and focused information about a patient. The use of the tool is advocated to enhance communication between individuals within clinical settings; it provides structure for an interaction, helping the individual giving information and those receiving it by ensuring the giver has formulated their thinking before trying to communicate it to someone else. (For further information on the SBAR tool, please see the useful websites at the end of this chapter.)

Now consider how this referral should be made using SBAR, within the following activity.

Activity 4.3   Inter-professional and team working

Make notes as to how you would complete an SBAR for referring Mrs Patel to the Critical Care Outreach Team.

An outline answer is given at the end of the chapter.

Having explored assessment of Mrs Patel, we will now move on to the immediate management.

Immediate management

The priorities of care for Mrs Patel relate to reperfusion, pain relief, vasodilation and oxygenation, which this section will now explore.

Usually, pharmacological interventions are given first as they are easily accessible when compared with procedures such as reperfusion therapy; however, clinical assessment for eligibility for reperfusion therapy should be a priority (NICE, 2020a).

Reperfusion therapy

Patients who present with a STEMI should receive 'reperfusion therapy' within 12 hours of symptom onset. Cardiac reperfusion therapy is a treatment that aims to restore the flow of blood within the heart by removing the blockage within the blood vessel.

This procedure, known as a percutaneous coronary intervention (PCI), is performed under X-ray, whereby an interventional radiologist finds the blocked vessel and removes it with a catheter that is entered through either the radial or femoral artery. In a situation where a PCI is not available, thrombolysis may be a treatment choice. Thrombolysis is a treatment whereby drugs are given to the patient to help break down the clot within the coronary arteries.

Pain relief

It is essential that Mrs Patel is made as comfortable as possible. If patients are in pain this can often place the heart under further strain. Intravenous opiates such as morphine are often recommended as a first line treatment for patients who are suffering with chest pain.

Vasodilation (widening of blood vessels)

Another course of treatment is to administer glycerine trinitrate (GTN), as this will cause vasodilation (widening of the blood vessels within the heart) and therefore allow for more blood to get to the heart muscle and often also relieve pain for some patients.

Oxygen

The administration of oxygen should be avoided in patients who are presenting with STEMI if the oxygen saturation is above 94 per cent or 88–92 per cent or for those patients who have type 2 respiratory failure. The administration of oxygen can cause vasoconstriction and therefore result in a further reduction of blood flow to the heart muscle. However, for those patients who have oxygen saturation below the expected levels, supplementary oxygen should be prescribed and administered until the desired saturation level has been reached.

To conclude looking at assessment, when assessing Mrs Patel a systematic approach such as the ABCDE assessment should be used. You will also need to document other findings such as a pain assessment. Any patients who report chest pain should have a comprehensive assessment completed by an RN and this should be escalated appropriately depending on the findings of the assessment.

Following cardiac assessment and immediate management, it is important to ensure ongoing care and medication management is then addressed.

Ongoing care of Mrs Patel

Mrs Patel has been informed at the bedside that she is currently having a myocardial infarction; this will require the patient to have constant monitoring and assessment for suitability for reperfusion therapy by a senior member of the medical team. This would need to have been completed within 90 minutes of diagnosis within a hospital setting if she is deemed eligible. You may be asked to gather equipment together, such as the resuscitation trolley, in case it is required. Constant monitoring and recording of observations will be required using an ABCDE approach. You should consider placing the patient on a 3-lead ECG to identify any life-threatening arrhythmias.

A major priority for treatment is to control her pain; increased levels of pain will place her heart under further strain. As a NA you may be asked by the RN to complete a pain assessment to develop a full understanding of her pain level and the type of pain she is in. Mrs Patel can be given IV morphine to relieve her pain, and can be placed in a semi-recumbent position as this is often the most comfortable position for patients who have chest pain.

Mrs Patel is likely to be prescribed aspirin to stop the clot becoming larger, GTN to create vasodilation and increase blood flow to the myocardium and clopidogrel to further reduce clot formation.

Mrs Patel has compromised cardiac functioning and needs to have strict fluid balance monitored – this may require a urinary catheter to be inserted.

Mrs Patel will need to be transferred to an area that can deliver critical care interventions; this would likely be intensive care or a coronary care unit. Other investigations such as blood tests may also be required, depending on local policy.

Longer term care

Following a cardiac event or cardiac surgery, all patients should enter a structured process known as cardiac rehabilitation. It allows for patients with heart disease to achieve a healthier lifestyle and has been found to reduce cardiac deaths by over 25 per cent (British Heart Foundation, 2018). As an NA you may work within a cardiac rehabilitation service or be involved with the referral of a patient such as Mrs Patel, who has had a STEMI.

Cardiac rehabilitation gives patients as well as their families information, support and advice on how to ensure that they can remain in good health and prevent further cardiac events in the future. Patients will have an individualised plan that is made up of exercises and educational sessions to complete, following discharge from hospital. This may be delivered within a patient's own home or at a cardiac rehabilitation centre and may also take place in a local leisure centre or hospital. Patients would usually attend two sessions a week. Programmes will usually last for up to 10–12 weeks with each session lasting around two hours.

Chapter summary

This chapter has outlined the assessment and management of a patient with a STEMI, focused on a case study, Mrs Patel, who developed a STEMI within a ward setting. As an NA or NA student it is important that you understand the cardiac anatomy, physiology and pathophysiology in order to provide effective evidence-based care. The assessment of a patient with a STEMI requires a number of components which have been explored. The immediate priorities of care have been identified, along with ongoing and longer-term care.

Activities: brief outline answers

Activity 4.1: Critical thinking

Below is an outline of the abnormal observations:

Respiratory rate: 23
The respiratory rate is elevated, a normal respiratory rate should be between 12 and 20

Blood pressure: 160/96
The blood pressure is elevated, a blood pressure above a systolic of 140mmHg would be deemed as hypertension

Pulse: 106
The pulse is elevated, a pulse above 90 would be deemed as tachycardia.

The observations along with the presentation of Mrs Patel should be of concern to you as a NA. The observations are likely to be abnormal because of heart ischemia and pain. It would be expected that you escalate this patient immediately to the RN allocated to the patient and possibly senior medical team members.

Immediate concerns: chest pain, clammy skin, and the possibility of this patient deteriorating.

Activity 4.2 Evidence-based practice and research

Mrs Patel has diabetes, which increases the risks of developing CHD, particularly when this is uncontrolled. It's important that all patients with diabetes have education to ensure that their blood sugar levels are controlled.

Mrs Patel is of South Indian heritage, and this also increases the risk of her developing CHD. This is thought to be because of the increased risk of diabetes as well as body shape (central obesity).

Mrs Patel requires assistance with her activities of daily living (ADLs) and has very little exercise – both factors mean that she is likely to have an increased risk of developing CHD.

Activity 4.3 Inter-professional and team working

Situation

Hello my name is ... I am an NA working on the cardiac ward.

I am calling about Mrs Patel in bed ...

I am calling for a referral to your services as she has ST elevation on her ECG, the medical team are already in the bed space.

Mrs Patel is a 62-year-old female who has been admitted onto the cardiac ward for investigation of chest pain. She was admitted after reporting a seven-day history of increasing fatigue and shortness of breath on exertion; she reports that she has had the chest pain for three days.

Background

Mrs Patel is of South Asian heritage, has type-II diabetes which is uncontrolled and has peripheral vascular disease. She relies on her family to complete her activities of daily living. Mrs Patel has awoken this morning and has complained of increasing chest pain; she is also clammy.

Assessment

Airway:
Patent but unable to converse in full sentences.

Breathing:
Respiratory rate – 23
Oxygen saturation – 96%
She is currently on room air
Circulation:
Blood pressure: 160/90
Pulse: 106
ECG: has been completed and the patient is connected to a cardiac monitor
CRT: 4 seconds
Disability:
Consciousness: alert
Exposure:
Temperature: 36.2

Recommendation

The medical team are already in the bed space, and I have informed the nurse in charge. Would you please be able to come and review this patient?

Further reading

Waugh, A. and Grant, A. (2022) *Ross & Wilson Anatomy and Physiology in Health and Illness*. E-Book. London: Elsevier.

This book is clear and unambiguous when it comes to explaining anatomy and physiology. The chapter on the cardiovascular system explains the anatomy of the heart well, as well as the pathophysiology of the disease process for conditions such as atherosclerosis.

Useful websites

www.youtube.com/watch?v=TBG9Jw3yd9I

Acute Coronary Syndrome Detailed Overview (MI, STEMI, NSTEMI). This YouTube video gives a detailed overview of acute coronary syndromes including a STEMI. The video explains the pathophysiology as well as the investigations required to treat patients that present with a STEMI.

www.nice.org.uk/guidance/ng185

The NICE guideline for acute coronary syndromes explains in detail the early and longer-term management of patients who have an acute coronary syndrome. The guideline aims to improve survival and quality of life for patients who have a myocardial infarction or unstable angina.

www.england.nhs.uk/wp-content/uploads/2021/03/qsir-sbar-communication-tool.pdf

SBAR tool

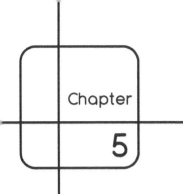

Chapter 5

The acutely ill neurological patient: ischemic stroke

Laura Whitehead

(Continued)

3.15 understand the principles of safe and effective administration and optimisation of medicines in accordance with local and national policies

3.16 demonstrate the ability to recognise the effects of medicines, allergies, drug sensitivity, side effects, contraindications and adverse reactions

Chapter aims

By the end of this chapter you should be able to:

- define what is meant by the term stroke and the different types;
- explain the risk factors associated with stroke;
- understand how to assess a patient who is displaying signs of a stroke;
- discuss the management and monitoring that is required for a patient presenting with a stroke, including pharmacology;

Introduction

Stroke is defined by the World Health Organization (WHO) (2020, page 1) as a clinical syndrome consisting of 'rapidly developing clinical signs of focal (at times global) disturbance of cerebral function, lasting more than 24 hours or leading to death with no apparent cause other than that of vascular origin'. Worldwide strokes are the 'second leading cause of death and the third leading cause of disability' (WHO, 2020, page 1). Strokes are one of the leading causes of death in the UK (Stroke Association, 2020). Strokes are also a leading cause of dementia and depression. Every five minutes in the United Kingdom an adult has a stroke. A stroke is a type of cerebrovascular disease, a term used to describe anything that affects blood flow to the brain. When a person has a stroke, it causes the sudden death of brain cells due to a lack of oxygen. This occurs when there is a reduction in the blood flow to the brain due to a blockage or a rupture of an artery.

The Stroke Association UK collate and publish data every year around the prevalence of strokes and patient outcomes in their report *State of the Nation* (2020). From this report, it is estimated that around 100,000 people every year suffer from a stroke, and there are 1.3 million stroke survivors currently in the UK. Around 25–33 per cent are recurrent strokes; normally people can survive a first stroke, but approximately two thirds of stroke survivors leave hospital with some form of a disability (Stroke Association, 2020). This can mean that over a third of people who have suffered from a stroke will be dependent on others for assistance with carrying out their daily activities (NICE, 2019a). Stroke survivors can experience significant on-going medical problems that include the possibility of having a recurrent stroke, transient ischaemic attacks (TIAs) and/or death (Stroke Association, 2018).

In 2007 the National Stroke Strategy was published by the Department of Health. The aim was to produce a national framework which would improve stroke care over the next ten years

(DOH, 2007). One of the main changes to stroke care was the development of Hyper Acute Stroke Units (HASUs), to ensure that anyone suffering from a stroke could be treated rapidly by expert multidisciplinary teams (DOH, 2007). Following the publication of the National Stroke Strategy, care of the stoke patient has been an essential feature in the NHS Long Term Plan 2021. A standardised stroke care pathway combines hospital, community and rehabilitation care of the stroke patient (NHS England, 2021b).

A full care pathway was introduced to ensure continuity of care from the community, hospital and rehabilitation community care (NHS England, 2021b), the aim being to save half a million lives over the next decade and improve the recovery of hundreds of thousands of people (NHS England, 2021b).

This chapter will outline the different types of stroke and will provide you with the necessary pathophysiology knowledge needed to assess and care for patients presenting with a stroke. The chapter will focus on ischemic strokes in detail, using a case study and self-directed activities. This chapter will use a rolling case study, where information about the patient will be presented at various stages, such as admission, A&E and post intervention. You will be guided through the assessment of a stroke patient, learn how to identify nursing problems and implement nursing management of a patient presenting with a stroke. There are model answers provided at the end of the chapter for you to utilise once you have completed the activities.

Case study: Anisha, the acutely ill neurological patient

Anisha is a 60-year-old woman, with a past medical history of high cholesterol, which is being treated with atorvastatin 20mg once a day (OD); she is also overweight with a BMI of 25. Anisha works full time as a teacher and is independent in all of her activities in daily living (Roper, Logan and Tiernay, 2000). She is a member of her local choir and leads a very busy life, which means she exercises less then she would like to and eats takeaways three times a week whilst she is working late. Whilst teaching a lesson at work, a pupil noticed that Anisha's speech became slurred and she had some facial drooping to the left side.

Pathophysiology of the brain

Blood is supplied to the brain by two major blood vessels (Peate and Dutton, 2012). The anterior circulation comes from the right and left internal carotid arteries and the posterior circulation is from the two vertebral arteries (Goulden and Clarke, 2016). These form a structure called a circle of Willis (see Figure 5.1) and are connected to the base of the brain (Goulden and Clarke, 2016). The circle of Willis supplies most of the brain with blood, and it also equalises blood pressure throughout the brain. It can also provide an alternative blood supply if an artery in the brain becomes blocked (Peate and Dutton, 2012). Loss of blood flow to the brain results in the brain lacking the oxygen its cells require to function and causes irreversible damage to the brain (Peate and Dutton, 2012).

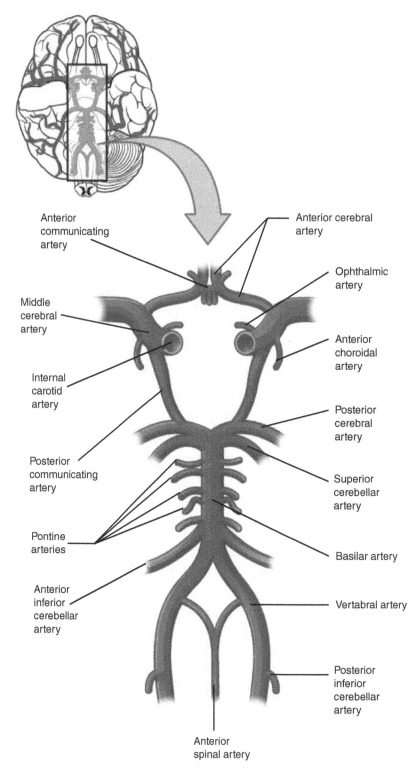

Figure 5.1 Circle of Willis (© Openstax)

Structure of the brain

The brain and spinal cord are protected by key structures. As shown in Figure 5.2, these include bone that surrounds the spinal cord and the cranium (the brain), the meninges, cerebrospinal fluid, the blood–brain barrier (Boore et al., 2016). The meninges are made up of three layers of connective tissue, the dura matter, pia matter and subarachnoid space (Boore et al., 2016).

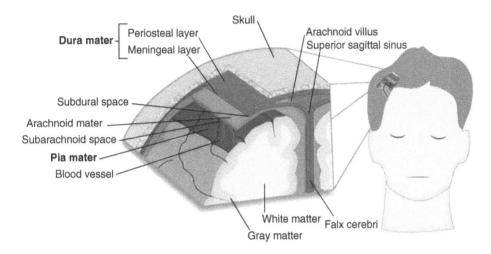

Figure 5.2   The meninges (Cook, 2021)

Function of the brain

Each area of the brain has a particular function (Puthenpurakal and Crussell, 2017). Look at Figure 5.3 below and look at the different names and parts of the brain. Figure 5.3 also includes information about the function. Stroke patients will present with different symptoms depending on what area of the brain is affected.

Types of stroke

There are three main types of stroke: transient ischemic attack, haemorrhagic and ischemic.

Transient Ischemic Attack

A transient ischemic attack (TIA) is a temporary reduction in blood flow to the brain. The blood clot and resulting symptoms only last for a short period of time. This may be called a mini stroke or a warning stroke (Barclay and Jones, 2018). The risk for developing an acute stroke is at its greatest in the first few days after a TIA. Patients who have had a TIA need to be seen by a specialist so further imaging and medications can be discussed (NICE, 2019a). TIAs are caused by blood clots, either due to the patient being in atrial fibrillation, a clot forming and travelling to the brain or due to damage in the carotid arteries in the neck caused by atherosclerosis (Barclay and Jones, 2018). These risk factors and cause of TIA will be discussed later on in the chapter.

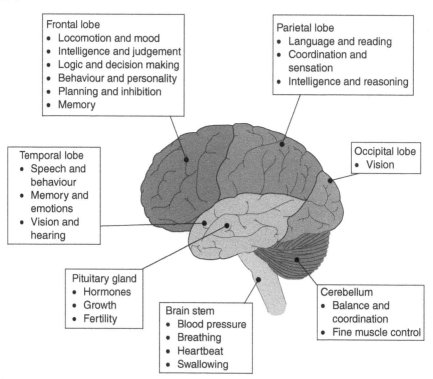

Figure 5.3 Areas of the brain and their functions (adapted from Cook, 2021)

Haemorrhagic stroke

A haemorrhagic stroke is due to bleeding in or around the brain. There are two main types of haemorrhagic stroke: intracerebral/intracranial, or subarachnoid haemorrhage. An intracerebral/intracranial haemorrhage (ICH) occurs as a result of bleeding within lobes, pons or cerebellum of the brain (Clarke and Beaumont, 2016). The bleed happens in the brain tissue itself. Subarachnoid haemorrhage (SAH) is when the bleed happens between the arachnoid membrane and the pia matter (Markus et al., 2010). A SAH occurs when the blood vessels on the surface of the brain burst and blood leaks into the subarachnoid space (Markus et al, 2010). Around 10 per cent of haemorrhagic strokes are due to a SAH, the most common cause being a burst aneurysm (Stroke Association, 2020).

A haemorrhagic stroke occurs when a weakened blood vessel ruptures (Markus et al., 2010). This weakness may be due to an aneurysm, arteriovenous malformations, high blood pressure or drug use. High blood pressure (hypertension) can damage vessels in the brain and makes them more prone to bleeding (Stroke Association, 2020). Cerebral amyloid angiopathy (CAA) is a type of small vessel disease where a protein called amyloid building up within a small blood vessel can damage the vessel and cause it to tear and bleed (Stroke Association, 2020). CAA is common in older people and people with dementia (Stroke Association, 2020). Micro bleeds are very common in people with CAA; they may not present with any symptoms but the bleeds are apparent on a scan of the patient's brain.

An aneurysm bursting is also a cause of a haemorrhagic stroke. An aneurysm is caused when a weak spot in an artery balloons out and becomes stretched (Peate and Dutton, 2012). Aneurysms most commonly occur in the abdominal aorta and the brain (Peate and Dutton, 2012). Some people have aneurysm from birth; however, there are other risk factors including high blood pressure, smoking, family history of them, using cocaine and a genetic kidney condition called autosomal dominant polycystic kidney disease (Stroke Association, 2020).

Very rarely some people may be born with blood vessel malformations, which is where blood vessels can be enlarged and be in clusters (Zyck and Gould, 2021). Cavernous malformation is a type of vessel malformation where the vessel walls are thin and can cause bleeds in the brain (Zyck and Gould, 2021).

Ischemic Stroke

Approximately 85 per cent of strokes are ischemic (Stroke Association, 2020). In an ischemic stroke a blockage cuts off the blood supply to the brain. This blockage can be caused by a blood clot located in an artery or blood vessels within the brain; commonly this occurs in the carotid artery (Stroke Association, 2020).

A blood clot can form due to a variety of reasons, such as:

- *atherosclerosis* – is when fatty deposits build up in the walls of the large and medium sized arteries (Malecki-Ketchell, 2016). These fatty deposits can cause the artery to become harder and narrower, which increases the likelihood of arteries becoming occluded (Malecki-Ketchell, 2016). Atherosclerosis can occur with age, or due to lifestyle factors such as smoking, unhealthy foods, lack of exercise or medical conditions like high blood pressure, high cholesterol or diabetes (Malecki-Ketchell, 2016). Atherosclerosis can occur in any artery within the body, particularly the carotid arteries, which are in the neck and supply the brain with blood. The fatty deposits within these arteries can break off and form a clot, which can block the artery or travel in the blood stream and block an artery in the brain (Stroke Association, 2020) (see Figure 4.7 in Chapter 4 for a diagram showing the development of an atheroma);
- *small vessel disease* – where there is damage to the smaller blood vessels within the brain. This leads to reduced blood flow and causes damage to the brain cells as they are not getting enough oxygen or glucose. The main risk factor for this damage is high blood pressure and it can lead to conditions like vascular dementia;
- *atrial fibrillation* – is a heart condition where the heart beats irregularly and leads to an increased risk of embolisms. These blood clots can move in the blood stream and to the brain.

This is not an exhaustive list, and there are a number of other factors that can contribute to a person having a stroke. It is important that when any patient presents with signs and symptoms of a stroke (and when it is safe to do so), a comprehensive past medical history must be established.

Activity 5.1   Critical thinking

Using the information within this chapter and from your own reading, list the risk factors associated with ischemic strokes and identify what factors make Anisha at high risk of an ischemic stroke.

- What about her lifestyle makes her high risk?
- What about her past medical history makes her have a higher risk of developing an ischemic stroke?

An outline answer is given at the end of the chapter.

Recognising the signs of stroke

Recognising the signs of a stroke is key to ensuring the patient receives timely treatment. The medical, surgical and pharmacological interventions used to treat patients who have had a stroke are only effective if they are given within a certain time frame. Timely treatment helps improve a patient's chances of recovery (NICE, 2020c). One of the most widely known stroke recognition and action tools used in the United Kingdom is the algorithm facial weakness, arm weakness, speech problems and time (FAST) (Department of Health, 2009):

- *facial weakness*: can the person smile? Is there any new drooping of their mouth, lips or eyes?
- *arm weakness*: can the person raise both of their arms? Is there any new difference in their left or right arm?
- *speech problems*: can the person speak clearly? Can they be understood?
- *time to call 999*: if the person is experiencing any of these signs.

The FAST test is a quick way of assessing the most common signs and symptoms of a stroke.

FAST can also be used to assess patients presenting with the following signs and symptoms:

- sudden weakness or numbness on one side of the body, including legs, hands or feet;
- difficulty finding words or speaking in clear sentences;
- sudden blurred vision or loss of sight in one or both eyes;
- sudden memory loss or confusion, and dizziness or a sudden fall;
- a sudden, severe headache.

If you notice any of these symptoms this needs to be treated as an emergency (Department of Health, 2009). (For further information in relation to the FAST assessment, please see the video created by UK Health Security Agency (2015) in the useful websites section at the end of this chapter.)

We will now be exploring the actions of a student NA in the context of Anisha, our patient who was discussed in the case study earlier in the chapter.

Activity 5.2   Reflection

Urgent medical care is essential in treating patients presenting with a stroke. Answering the following reflective questions will help you appreciate that seeking urgent medical attention is essential for survival following a stroke:

1.   Why is it important to call an ambulance straight away when a person shows sudden onset of facial/arm weakness or slurred speech?
2.   If the person showing the above signs was in hospital, what would you as a student NA do?

An outline answer is given at the end of the chapter

Case study: Anisha (continued)

An ambulance was immediately called and Anisha was taken by paramedics to a hospital which has a Hyper Acute Stroke Unit. In the ambulance Anisha's facial drooping became worse and her speech remained slurred. She was alert throughout (we will be discussing assessing a patient's level of consciousness later on in the chapter). The paramedic performed a set of vital signs and discovered: blood pressure 165/80mmHg, heart rate of 88 beats per minute, temperature of 36.5 °C, oxygen saturation 97 per cent with a respiratory rate 18 breaths per minute.

Anisha was taken to the Resuscitation area within A&E and assessed by a registered nurse (RN) and student nursing associate (NA). Upon arriving at A&E Anisha was taken for a head computerised tomography (CT) scan. The CT head scan showed that Anisha had a blocked blood vessel in her brain and she was diagnosed with an ischemic stroke. The stroke medical team were called to come and assess Anisha as a matter of urgency.

Assessing Anisha, the stroke patient

The registered nurse and the student nursing associate will now undertake an ABCDE assessment (RCUK, 2021b) on Anisha, which we also explored in Chapter 3. This assessment is carried out on all deteriorating or critically ill patients. The aim is to identify and treat any life-threatening problems and to work out whether the treatment provided is having the desired effect. It is vital that throughout this assessment patient consent is gained (Nursing and Midwifery Council, 2018d). The patient privacy must be maintained and their dignity and respect must be upheld (NMC, 2018d):

Airway – is the patient able to maintain their own airway? Is the airway clear? If the patient is able to talk this means there is no obstruction. Use the look, listen, feel approach – are there any foreign bodies like vomit or blood in the patient's airway? Can you hear any noises? Snoring is a sign of an obstructed airway; you would need to get expert help as soon as possible in this situation. The patient would need to be put on their side or a 'chin lift' would need to be performed to move the tongue out of the way. Feel – is there air moving in and out of the mouth? (RCUK, 2021b).

It was decided that Anisha could maintain her own airway and was able to speak.

Breathing – use the look, listen and feel approach. Is the patient showing any signs of distress – sweating, central cyanosis (blue lips) or peripheral cyanosis (blue tinged fingers or nails)? Does the patient look like they are having to work hard to breathe (high work of breathing)? Is the patient's breathing deep or shallow? What is their respiratory rate? What is the patient's oxygen saturation? If they are below 96 per cent or below 88–92 per cent in patients with respiratory conditions, such as chronic obstructive pulmonary disorder, then oxygen will need to be administered.

Anisha was showing no signs of respiratory distress, her oxygen saturation and respiratory rate were normal.

Circulation – what is the patient's heart rate? They should be attached to a cardiac monitor. The patient's capillary refill time (CRT) should be assessed by applying pressure for 5 seconds to the patient's fingertip held at heart level. The normal CRT is less than 2 seconds; if it takes longer for the skin to return to the colour of the surrounding skin this is a sign of poor peripheral perfusion. What is the patient's blood pressure? Temperature via a tympanic? What is the patient's urine output (the aim is 0.5mls/kg/hr)? If Anisha weighs 85kg then her target urine output would be 42.5mls an hour.

Disability – what is the patient's level of consciousness? What is their Glasgow Coma score (Teasdale, 2014) (this will be discussed later on in the chapter). Are their pupils equal? What size are they? Are they reactive to light? (Pupillary assessment will be discussed further on in the chapter.) What is the patient's blood glucose level? Are they in any pain? Are there any neurological symptoms?

Anisha is opening her eyes spontaneously, she is orientated and is able to obey commands. She does have slurred speech. She denies feeling any pain. The blood glucose aim for people suffering from acute stroke is 4 and 11 mmol/litre (NICE, 2019). Her capillary blood glucose is 7mmol/L.

Exposure – are the patient's pressure areas intact? Are they at risk of a pressure injury? What is their Waterlow score (Waterlow, 2005)? Are there any wounds/sores/bruises/scratches? Are there any invasive devices present? Are these documented?

Within the disability section you conducted a neurological assessment of Anisha; this will now be discussed in further detail.

Neurological assessment

It is vital as a student NA that you are able to conduct a neurological assessment. You might be very familiar with the ACVPU assessment tool, which is part of the National Early Warning Score (RCP, 2017). ACVPU enables a rapid neurological assessment. The acronym stands for alert, confusion (new onset), voice, pain or unresponsive. The assessment tool was updated in 2017 to include C for confusion, which is for any patients with new onset confusion or reduction in their GCS or delirium which could be due to suspected or confirmed sepsis (RCP, 2017). It is important that all healthcare professionals who are carrying out a NEWS assessment are training in its components and are able to record and act on the results obtained (RCP, 2017). You may also be familiar with the Glasgow Coma Scale (Teasdale, 2014), which is an in-depth assessment tool for neurological assessment.

Assessing Anisha using the Glasgow Coma Scale

The Glasgow Coma Scale, or GCS, was originally developed by Teasdale and Jennett in 1974 as a tool that can be used to communicate about the level of consciousness of patients with a brain injury. Now the assessment tool is used for all patients, as a way of monitoring and assessing their level of consciousness.

The assessment uses a scoring system made up of three components (Teasdale, 2014) – eyes, verbal and motor. It also includes a pupillary assessment, which will be discussed later on in the chapter. Each of the three components is given a score out of 15. Best eye opening gets a maximum 4 points, best verbal response gets a maximum 5 points and best motor response gets a maximum 6 points. These scores are then added together; the total score can range between 3/15, which is the lowest you can score, and 15/15, which is the highest.

Anisha is currently opening her eyes spontaneously, she is orientated to time, place and person and she is obeying commands; this means her GCS is 15/15.

It is important that you use the best level of response seen for each component.

Table 5.1 Glasgow Coma Scale (adapted from Teasdale, 2014)

Eyes	Verbal	Motor
Spontaneous (4)	Orientated (5)	Obeys commands (6)
To sound (3)	Confused (4)	Localising (5)
To pressure (2)	Words (3)	Normal flexion (4)
None (1)	Sounds (2)	Abnormal flexion (3)
	None (1)	Extension (2)
		None (1)

Activity 5.3   Critical thinking

Now please access the Glasgow Coma Score assessment aid via the website provided and answer the following questions:

Teasdale (2014) Glasgow Coma Scale website: www.glasgowcomascale.org/downloads/GCS-Assessment-Aid-English.pdf?v=3

- What does it mean when a patient's eyes are open spontaneously?
- What 'pressure' are they referring to? What do healthcare professionals have to be mindful of when using pressure to assess a person's response?
- What does a person have to be orientated to in order to be awarded a 5?
- What is an example of a command you could give a patient in order to assess a person's motor function?

An outline answer is given at the end of the chapter.

Conducting a pupillary assessment on Anisha

Assessing the patient's pupils is a vital part of the GCS assessment (Teasdale, 2014). Any changes in the pupils' shape, size and ability to react provides important information about what is going on in the patient's brain. Pupils should be the same size and shape, although if the patient has had cataract or other eye surgery this may not be the case (Teasdale, 2014). You should also ask if the patient has ever had any eye injuries or if they have a glass eye. It is important that you take into consideration the patient's past medical history when undertaking any assessment (Teasdale, 2014). It is also important you know what medication the patient is taking; for example topical beta-blockers and opioids can cause pupillary constriction (Teasdale, 2014).

Anisha's pupils have been assessed. They are equal in size and are a size 3. They are reactive to light. She does not have any previous eye injuries and is not on any medication which would impact pupillary response.

Pathophysiology of the eye

The pupil is the black circle in the centre of the iris (the coloured area of the eye) (Marcovitch, 2005). The pupil should constrict, i.e. get smaller as a response to bright light stimulus. In darkness the pupil should dilate (become bigger). The size of the pupil changes when the muscles in the iris contract and relax (Marcovitch, 2005). These are controlled by the oculomotor nerve. The oculomotor nerve is the third cranial nerve and by assessing the pupillary reaction, we are assessing this nerve (Marcovitch, 2005). If this nerve is compressed this results in the pupils becoming fixed – they will not respond to light stimulus and they will be dilated (Marcovitch, 2005). If a person has any change in their level of consciousness, their GCS and then a pupillary assessment must be done as a matter of urgency (Teasdale, 2014). This is because any changes in the pupillary response, size or shape, along with any changes in GCS, are a sign that the patient has an increase in the amount of pressure in their brain. This can be due to a stroke or as a result of trauma (Teasdale, 2014). This is considered a medical emergency and should be treated as such.

Assessing Anisha's pupil size and shape

Pupils should respond briskly (quickly) to bright light (Jevon, 2007). They might respond sluggishly or even not all. It is important that the reaction is documented and communicated with other members of the multidisciplinary team (Jevon, 2007). Pen torches are available in most clinical areas; it is important that you also have a pupil size guide present when carrying out your assessment. As discussed earlier, if pupils do not react, this is a sign of increased pressure in the brain and is a medical emergency.

Prior to carrying out the assessment you should explain the procedure to the patient (NMC, 2018d), regardless of their level of consciousness. Consent should be gained prior to any assessment or intervention (NMC, 2018d). Ensure that you have washed your hands and are adhering to the personal protective equipment guidance (NHS England, 2020). If possible, dim the overhead light; however, due to the clinical areas this may not be possible. Using the pupil sizing chart, assess the patient's pupil size. Compare their size and shape. After you have warned the patient, shine the torch into the patient's eye. You are looking to see whether there is a response and at what speed it occurs. Do this for both eyes. Once you have assessed the response in each eye, you are now going to shine the light into each eye whilst looking at the opposite pupil. You are looking to see whether the opposite pupil constricts – this is called the consensual response (Jevon, 2007). Carry out the same procedure for the other eye. Ensure that this information is documented in the patient's notes.

If there are any changes or deterioration this needs to be communicated as a matter of urgency to the nurse in charge and to the medical team (NMC, 2018d). Patients who have had a stroke, like Anisha, can deteriorate, which may manifest itself in changes to her pupillary reaction; therefore regular assessments need to be conducted.

Case study: Anisha (continued)

On arrival back from CT, Anisha's blood pressure is 170/80mmHg, heart rate 90 beats per minute (bpm) sinus tachycardia, apyrexic with a temperature of 37 °C, oxygen saturation of 97 per cent on room air and a respiratory rate of 19. Anisha weighs 85kg and passed 50mls of urine in the commode. Her capillary blood glucose is 10mmol/L. Her Glasgow Coma Score is 15/15 (Teasdale and Jennett, 1974). Her pupils are equal and briskly reactive to light. They are both 4mm in size.

Activity 5.4   Evidence-based practice

Using the information from the case study, the ABCDE assessment (RCUK, 2021b) you have conducted and the vital signs above, what are two nursing problems that you have identified?

Now compare what you have written with the model answer at the end of the chapter. Are the answers correct?

Reflect on the work you have completed. Were there areas or issues identified that you did not consider?

An outline answer is given at the end of the chapter.

Management of Anisha's ischemic stroke

This section will focus on the management of an ischemic stroke and will discuss the pharmacological interventions that are part of the plan of care for Anisha. The stroke medical team decided that as the onset of her symptoms prior to the CT was < 1.5 hours, Anisha was suitable for thrombolysis treatment Alteplase (NICE, 2019a). Alteplase must be started as soon as possible, within 4.5 hours of the start of the stroke symptoms, a CT head scan should be carried out to rule out an intracranial haemorrhage (bleed in the brain) (NICE, 2019a). As per the British National Formulary (BNF, 2021b) the Registrar has prescribed 900/micrograms/per kg. Anisha weighs 85kg and has been prescribed a dose of 76.5mg. The registered nurse prepares the intravenous medication and administers it over 60 minutes (BNF, 2021b).

Pharmacology

Alteplase is a fibrinolytic drug. This means it activates plasminogen to form plasmin. This plasmin then breaks down fibrin, which breaks up the thrombi (the clot) (BNF, 2021b). Anisha must be monitored continuously for signs of bleeding, changes in her blood pressure, level of consciousness and pupils.

Activity 5.5   Evidence-based practice

Consider how you as a student nursing associate would monitor Anisha.

- What equipment would you use?
- What assessment tools would you use to assess her?

Anisha's systolic blood pressure must be below 180mmHg and her diastolic below 105mmHg.

(Continued)

(Continued)

- Using the information from the scenario above, is Anisha's blood pressure within this target range?
- Is any intervention required?

An outline answer is given at the end of the chapter.

NICE (2019a), in the report *Stroke and TIA in over 16s: diagnosis and management*, outline the importance of starting aspirin 300mg daily, either orally or via an enteral tube if the patient has issues swallowing. This should be reviewed after two weeks, as the patient would need to be on an antithrombotic treatment.

Other medications

Aspirin, or *acetylsalicylic acid* is a non-steroidal anti-inflammatory; however it also inhibits normal platelet function. Anisha would continue her daily dose of atorvastatin 20mg (NICE, 2019a).

Case study: Anisha (continued)

Anisha was transferred to the HASU ward, where she received close monitoring of her symptoms post alteplase infusion. Anisha was assessed by a speech and language therapist to ensure her ability to swallow had not been affected by the stroke. She was started on an early mobilisation programme and upon discharge was referred for community rehabilitation. Anisha recovered well from her stroke and after three months she was back at work teaching.

Chapter summary

This chapter has discussed in depth the care of a patient from when they first exhibited symptoms in the community, to the assessment and treatment in A&E and HASU. The case study has aided you in completing an ABCDE assessment of a patient exhibiting neurological symptoms, including a Glasgow Coma Scale assessment and an assessment of the pupillary response. You have identified nursing problems and how these would be prioritised. You have developed your pharmacology knowledge of the medications used in the treatment of an ischemic stroke. The model answers at the end of the chapter should be used to assist you in reflecting on the activities you have completed as you worked through this chapter.

Activities: brief outline answers

Activity 5.1 Critical thinking

Anisha has high cholesterol, a BMI of 25 and eats regular takeaways.

Activity 5.2 Reflection

The person with symptoms needs to be taken to a Hyper Acute Stroke Unit (HASU) as a matter of urgency. Some of the medications and interventions to treat patients who have had a stroke are only effective if they are given within a certain time frame. Timely treatment helps improve a patient's chances of recovery.

The ambulance needs to be called straightaway as the patient could be having a stroke.

Call for help, carry out an ABCDE assessment, contact the medical/surgical team as a matter of urgency; the patient would need a review from the stroke team.

Activity 5.3 Critical thinking

Examples of spontaneous eye opening: when a patient's eyes open immediately as you walk into the room, or when you call the patient's name.

Pressure can be fingertip touch or a trapezius squeeze if required. Must not exert unnecessary force, hurt or harm the patient in any way.

Patient has to be orientated to place, time and person in order to be awarded a 5 for verbal response.

You could ask the patient to stick their tongue out, lift their arm up and down, wiggle their toes. Ensure that the patient is capable of the action. A hand squeeze is a difficult action to assess as it could be an automatic response rather than a purposeful action.

Activity 5.4 Evidence-based practice

Risk of ineffective cerebral tissue perfusion/blood flow to the brain due to ischemic stroke as evidenced by slurred speech, altered level of consciousness, facial drooping and CT head scan report.

Impaired verbal communication due to ischemic stroke as evidenced by slurred speech and facial drooping.

Activity 5.5 Evidence-based practice

Monitor her vital signs; Anisha would be attached to continuous ECG monitoring, blood pressure cuff on 15-minute cycles, assessment tools – NEWS2, GCS/AVPU – Anisha's level of consciousness would be assessed along with her pupillary response.

Useful websites

www.stroke.org.uk/

The Stroke Association has a wide variety of information for professionals, patients and their families. Please utilise the resources on their website.

www.bhf.org.uk/informationsupport/conditions/stroke

The British Heart Foundation has evidence-based resources and information available on their website, particularly focused on cases, signs and symptoms.

www.youtube.com/watch?v=vc9OF64H4sE

The UK Health Security Agency (2015) provides further information in relation to the FAST assessment.

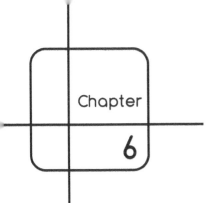

Chapter 6

The acutely ill endocrine patient: diabetic ketoacidosis

Tina Moore

NMC STANDARDS OF PROFICIENCY FOR NURSING ASSOCIATES

This chapter will address the following platforms and proficiencies:

Platform 3: Provide and monitor care

At the point of registration, the nursing associate will be able to:

3.2 demonstrate and apply knowledge of body systems and homeostasis, human anatomy and physiology, biology, genomics, pharmacology, social and behavioural sciences when delivering care

3.6 demonstrate the knowledge, skills and ability to perform a range of nursing procedures and manage devices, to meet people's need for safe, effective and person-centred care

3.7 demonstrate and apply an understanding of how and when to escalate to the appropriate professional for expert help and advice

3.11 demonstrate the ability to recognise when a person's condition has improved or deteriorated by undertaking health monitoring, interpret, promptly respond, share findings and escalate as needed

3.18 demonstrate the ability to monitor the effectiveness of care in partnership with people, families and carers. Document progress and report outcomes

Platform 4: Working in teams

At the point of registration, the nursing associate will be able to:

4.1 demonstrate an awareness of the roles, responsibilities and scope of practice of different members of the nursing and interdisciplinary team and their one role within it

4.9 discuss the influence of policy and political drivers that impact health and care provision

Chapter aims

After reading this chapter, you will be able to:

- understand how blood glucose is regulated in the body;
- identify the causes of diabetic ketoacidosis (DKA);
- demonstrate knowledge and understanding in relation to assessment and care management of DKA;
- consider health promotion strategies to minimise/prevent the occurrence of DKA.

Introduction

In the past, patients with diabetic ketoacidosis (DKA) would have been managed in a critical care environment (intensive care unit). This is no longer the case and today this type of patient is being cared for in general care areas. Depending on your work environment, you may have already been caring for patients who have a diagnosis of DKA. Alternatively, you may be exposed to such patients during other clinical placements during your nursing associate (NA) programme.

Within the UK, DKA is the leading cause of death amongst people under 58 years old with type 1 diabetes mellitus (Gibb et al., 2016). Therefore, specialist diabetic teams should be involved in the care of such patients as early as possible in order to increase the chances of a more favourable outcome (JBDS, 2021). Data suggests that the incidence of DKA ranges between 8.0 and 51.3 cases per 1000 adult patients (Farsani et al., 2017). This relates to those with type 1 diabetes, although DKA can also be seen in patients with type 2 diabetes. Likewise, there is a high cost associated with treating DKA. Estimates suggest for one occurrence this can be £2,064 (Desai et al., 2018).

High risk groups who have developed DKA have been identified as: the older person, pregnant woman, young people 18–25, those with heart or kidney failure or other serious comorbidities (JBDS, 2021). This targeted group will require diabetic specialist input as soon as possible and very careful monitoring of their illness, as their condition can deteriorate very quickly.

This chapter will focus on the adult, meaning those patients who are over the age of 18 years. Guidelines are slightly different for the child and young people, particularly around fluid replacement. If you are interested in learning more about this area, then you can find a suggestion in the further reading section at the end of the chapter. Within this chapter you will learn about the control of glucose within the body, understand the causes of DKA and the physiological reasons for presenting symptoms. The introduction of a case study will help you to systematically assess the patient's symptoms and identify their care needs. You will also learn about the management of a patient who is acutely ill with DKA. Discussions in particular around care management reflect current guidelines at the time of writing. First, this chapter will begin with a reflective and critical thinking activity as well as a case study.

Activity 6.1   Reflection

One of the fundamental physiological disturbances with patients who have DKA is the alterations to their blood glucose levels, leading to uncontrollable and high levels.

Depending on where you are in your NA programme, you may have had a number of different placements, you may have had only a few placements or you may not have commenced your placements as yet. Dependent upon the clinical setting of your work or placement area and the type of patients that you care for, you may have the task of monitoring patients' glucose levels.

Reflecting upon your experiences, think about the following questions:

- What were the reasons for monitoring the patient's blood glucose (e.g. were they diagnosed with diabetes? Were they receiving treatment that would increase their blood glucose levels, e.g. high doses of steroids? Were they critically ill? (The stress response during critical illness increases blood sugar levels.)
- How often were you recording blood glucose levels? In addition, were you monitoring the patient's ketone levels (blood or urine)? Depending upon your workplace, the testing of blood glucose may not be a task that the NA will be involved in but rather performed by the registered nurse (RN).
- What would you consider to be a normal blood glucose level?

As this activity is based on your own reflection, no outline answer is given at the end of this chapter.

This case study will be used throughout the chapter in order to help you to think about and understand a comprehensive and individualised approach to the care of a patient with DKA.

Case study: Veronica, the acutely ill endocrine patient

Veronica is an 18-year-old with type 1 diabetes mellitus. She was diagnosed three years ago. She has had several admissions to hospital with diabetic ketoacidosis (mainly for non-compliance). Recently she has been feeling unwell and has a two-day history of fever and sore throat. Veronica is admitted to the ward you are working on via A&E. Her visual appearance indicates dehydration, her skin is thin and dry, and her tongue is furred.

On admission she is semiconscious. The following observations were recorded:

- Glasgow Coma Scale: 12;
- pulse: 135 beats/minute;
- blood pressure: 88/55mmHg;
- respirations: 30/minute (Kussmaul breathing);

(Continued)

(Continued)

- oxygen saturation: 92% (on air);
- venous pH 7.31 (normal 7.35–7.45) and shows metabolic acidosis;
- urinalysis indicates ketones ++++ (ketonuria) and glucose ++ (glycosuria);
- blood glucose 28 mmol/L.

Her clinical symptoms and laboratory results confirm a diagnosis of diabetic ketoacidosis.

Activity 6.2   Critical Thinking

Answer the following questions before reading further:

- What is the function of blood glucose?
- How is glucose controlled within the body?
- What factors influence or interfere with the regulation of glucose?

An outline answer is provided at the end of this chapter.

Control of blood glucose (normal physiology)

Whilst Veronica has had several admissions regarding uncontrolled blood glucose levels, there have been numerous occasions where her glucose levels have been controlled successfully. The following discussion explains the normal physiology of blood glucose control.

The brain, renal medulla and erythrocyte (red blood cell) energy sources rely on glucose for normal functioning. The regulation of blood glucose is controlled by the pancreas. Hormones that are essential in the metabolism of carbohydrate and in the control of blood glucose are insulin and glucagon. Insulin and glucagon are hormones that are secreted by the islets of Langerhans within the pancreas. These islets of Langerhans are clusters of endocrine cells that secrete glucagon via the alpha cells and insulin via the beta cells. Their ability to function effectively will determine blood glucose levels. That is, hyperglycaemia (high blood glucose), hypoglycaemia (low blood glucose) or normal glucose levels (Waugh and Grant, 2018).

Carbohydrates and fats are broken down into smaller molecules by digestive enzymes. They are then absorbed into the bloodstream via the lymphatic system (causing a rise in blood concentration of glucose). Amino acids (a product of protein metabolism), fats and excess carbohydrates are stored as fat in the fat tissue or glycogen in the liver.

After a meal, glucose from the intestine is stored in the liver in the form of glycogen. By breaking down the glycogen stores in the liver and the production of new glucose, the blood glucose level is kept constant. For these changes to be made, insulin is necessary. Insulin is released by the rise or surge of blood glucose and promotes glucose uptake and production of proteins, carbohydrates and fats (also known as lipids).

When the blood glucose level is low, glucagon, growth hormone and catecholamines (epinephrine and norepinephrine) are circulated in the blood. Insulin binds to the plasma membrane of the target cell, increasing the permeability of the cell to glucose and resulting in an increased uptake of glucose. Extra glucose is stored as glycogen or converted to fat in the adipose tissue cell.

Therefore, the function of insulin is to prevent blood glucose levels from going too high by:

- promoting the transportation of glucose into the cells;
- promoting glycogen storage in the liver and muscle cells;
- converting glucose into fats and therefore inhibiting fat metabolism;
- promoting tissue growth by protein deposition.

The function of glucagon is to prevent blood glucose levels from going to low by:

- breaking down of triglycerides (stored fats) into fatty acids;
- glycogenolysis (breakdown of glycogen to glucose);
- gluconeogenesis (metabolic process of glucose production).

Figure 6.1 provides a summary of the process of blood glucose control.

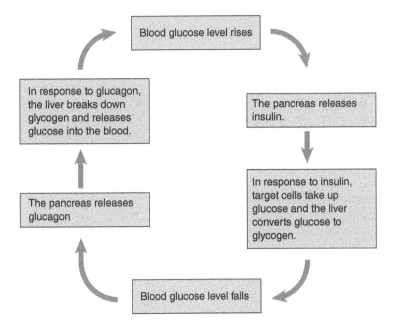

Figure 6.1   Summary of blood glucose control (© OpenStax)

Normal blood glucose levels are:

1. absent diagnosis of diabetes mellitus – 4.0 to 5.4 mmol/L;
2. diagnosis of diabetes mellitus – 4 to 7 mmol/L.

(Diabetes UK, 2021)

Diabetic ketoacidosis (DKA)

DKA is a common complication of diabetes mellitus, which mainly occurs in type 1 but can also occur in type 2. It results from severe deficiency of insulin, causing an altered metabolism of carbohydrates, proteins and fats. The outcomes of which are *hyperglycaemia* (high blood glucose level), *hyperosmolality* (high level of solute concentration in the blood), *ketoacidosis* (high level of blood acid (ketones)) and *volume depletion* (reduction in circulatory blood volume).

Patients suspected of having DKA should be appropriately and quickly assessed by observing for symptoms, for example, glycosuria (glucose in urine), ketonuria (ketones in urine) and hypotension (reduction in blood pressure), to confirm diagnosis. This is so that treatment can be started as soon as possible. The ability of healthcare professionals (including the NA) to recognise the clinical features of DKA profoundly affects outcome and survival rates (Hamdy, 2021).

DKA is considered to be a diabetic emergency and a potentially life-threatening condition. Symptoms can have a quick onset (over hours) or be more likely to be insidious and occur over the course of days. Irrespective of the time it takes for patients to demonstrate symptoms, fatal consequences can emerge, particularly if they are not identified quickly and treated appropriately and in a timely manner.

Criteria for the diagnosis of DKA includes all three of the following:

1. blood glucose of greater than 11.0mmol/l or known to have diabetes mellitus;
2. capillary/blood ketone – greater than 3.0 mmol/l or ketonuria (2+ or more);
3. venous pH – less than 7.3.

(JBDS, 2021)

Pathophysiology of DKA

DKA is a condition common amongst patients who are newly diagnosed with diabetes. Other causes of DKA can include anything that would initiate a physiological or psychological stress response (for the patient with diabetes or without diabetes); for example:

- an insult to the body, e.g. critical illness, undergoing extensive surgery, injury, sepsis, increasing age and concurrent illness such as infection – this may be a respiratory infection, or urinary tract infection;
- history of uncontrolled type 1 diabetes (or in some cases type 2 diabetes);
- accidental or deliberate omission of insulin (e.g. patients undergoing surgery or non-compliance).

The stress response relates to a cascade of metabolic and neurohormonal changes. Stress-induced hyperglycaemia is attributed to hypersecretion (increased secretion) of the counter regulatory hormones (catecholamines, glucagon, cortisol and growth hormone). Release of catecholamines results in decreased insulin and increased glucagon secretion by the pancreas. The effect is a surge in circulating glucose derived from glycogenolysis (breakdown of glycogen into glucose) and impaired utilisation of glucose (hyperglycaemia itself impairs glucose utilisation and residual insulin secretion).

It is helpful to apply your knowledge of physiology to the symptoms a patient will display; this is considered in the next activity.

Activity 6.3   Critical Thinking

From the case study, Veronica's symptoms can be categorised under four main headings:

- hyperglycaemia;
- dehydration;
- electrolyte loss;
- ketoacidosis.

Using these headings and from the information already provided, can you work out the symptoms that you would expect her to show? For example, she is dehydrated, so you would expect hypotension and tachycardia.

An outline answer is provided at the end of this chapter.

Clinical features of DKA

As DKA can provoke a life-threatening situation with fatal consequences, a thorough assessment of the patient is required. It is important to be extra vigilant when assessing the older person, as some symptoms may mimic other less acute conditions (JBDS, 2021). This presents an excellent opportunity to learn about developing your assessment skills and also the relationship between the body systems. In particular, the impact that one body system that is failing has on the functioning of other body systems. For example, a failing circulatory system (hypotension) will influence the performance of the renal system (causing a reduction in urine output). These will be discussed later in this chapter.

You are more likely to see the presentation of DKA in a secondary care area, particularly a hospital environment. However, DKA is a problem that could potentially occur at any time and in any place; even in a GP surgery or other primary care settings.

Clinical features of DKA include polyuria (increased volume of urine output), polydipsia (increased thirst), signs of metabolic acidosis (Kussmaul breathing), ketonuria. In the older patient, symptoms can be less overt. The main reason for this is that some symptoms may be equated to disorders of ageing and other diseases may mask symptoms, e.g. urinary frequency may be associated with prostatism in men (enlargement of the prostate causing obstruction at the neck of the bladder) or urinary tract infection in women. Kussmaul breathing may be mistaken for respiratory problems associated with severe heart failure or chest infection (Schwarzfuchs et al., 2020).

Observing for symptoms (such as glycosuria, ketonuria and hypotension) is required in order to confirm diagnosis and enable prompt intervention. Some of these may be new to you and are explored below.

1. *Hyperglycaemia*

Large volumes of water and electrolytes are lost due to osmotic diuresis (an increased serum osmolality that causes movement of water out of the cells and intracellular compartments leading to a depletion of fluid in these areas). As a result, dehydration occurs, which can result in a reduction in the level of consciousness. Counter regulatory hormones (discussed earlier) are released; these are broken down for energy (catabolic action), which further exacerbates hyperglycaemia. This in turn causes glycosuria.

2. *Glycosuria*

Glycosuria is also responsible for the loss of water through osmotic diuresis. In addition, glycosuria creates a favourable medium for the growth of yeast organisms; consequently, the patient may complain of pruritus (itching), particularly around the genitalia.

3. *Dehydration*

As discussed earlier, osmotic diuresis can cause considerable dehydration. Fluid is also lost through hyperventilation (fast breathing); vomiting; increased perspiration and decreased oral fluid intake. Polyuria can cause up to seven litres of free water to be lost (JBDS, 2021). Clinical signs include a dry mouth, dry skin and acute weight loss.

Compensatory mechanisms, stimulated by fluid volume depletion (in severe cases shock can occur), causes polydipsia (increased thirst). As a response, this action helps to maintain normal blood pressure.

4. *Electrolyte imbalances*

Electrolyte imbalances can result from the dehydration caused by polyuria. Sodium, potassium, phosphate and magnesium are all examples of electrolytes. Low blood concentrations of potassium, phosphate and magnesium can cause cardiac arrhythmias. If large volumes of fluid are given to the patient, their potassium levels may fall further. This is called haemodilution. Careful monitoring of the patient's potassium levels is essential.

5. *Ketonaemia (ketones in blood) and ketonuria*

Insulin deficiency prevents normal utilisation of serum glucose, leading to cellular starvation. The unmet energy requirements of the cells stimulate gluconeogenesis and glycogen conversion in the liver through the release of counter regulatory hormones. In the absence of glucose availability, the body is then forced to break down fat and protein stores to meet energy requirements. Ketone bodies (waste product of this process, called fat metabolism) accumulate in the blood, lowering the blood pH level (acidosis) (Waugh and Grant, 2018).

6. *Metabolic acidosis*

Metabolic acidosis is a clinical disturbance characterised by an increase in total body acid. In this case it is due to excessive lactic and keto acids occurring with a significant fall in plasma bicarbonate concentration and an imbalance in pH level. pH indicates whether the blood is acidic or alkaline in nature. Human blood is normally slightly alkaline.

Insulin deficiency prevents the normal utilisation of serum glucose, the outcome of which is starvation of the cells (even if there is an abundance of glucose in the blood, it cannot reach the cells). The unmet energy requirements of the cells stimulate gluconeogenesis and glycogen conversion in the liver through the release of counter regulatory hormones (previously discussed). Consequently, the body is forced to break down fat and protein stores to meet energy requirements. The rate of breakdown exceeds the body's ability to use these alternative energy sources. Ketone bodies accumulate in the blood, causing a lowering of the blood pH level, leading to metabolic acidosis.

Clinical presentations of metabolic acidosis include headache and lethargy. Severe acidosis can cause Kussmaul breathing (explained below), cardiac arrhythmias and eventually coma (JBDS, 2021). A low pH will stimulate the respiratory centre, producing an increased rate and depth of breathing. The odour of the breath generally smells fruity (this is the ketones).

7.   *Kussmaul breathing*

A low pH will trigger the respiratory centre to increase the rate and depth of breathing, in an attempt to 'blow off' carbon dioxide to compensate for acidosis. This is what is known as Kussmaul breathing.

8.   *General symptoms*

Classical symptoms include abdominal pain (usually generalised or epigastric). The abdomen may be rigid, with bowel sounds being irregular. Some symptoms may imitate gastrointestinal problems, causing diagnosis to be more difficult. The exact cause for this is still unknown. Other symptoms include nausea and vomiting.

Activity 6.4   Critical thinking

The criteria below indicate the symptoms of severe DKA. Revisit the case study and analyse Veronica's symptoms. Think about whether she is at risk of developing severe DKA. Think about providing a rationale for your answer.
   An outline answer is provided at the end of this chapter.

Severity of DKA

The severity of DKA is determined by the presence of one or more of the following (JBDS, 2021):

- blood ketones over 6.0 mmol/L;
- bicarbonate level below 5.0 mmol/L;
- venous/arterial pH below 7.0;
- hypokalaemia on admissions under 3.5 mmol/L;
- GCS $\geq$ 12 / abnormal AVPU;
- oxygen saturations $\leq$ 92% on air;
- systolic $\leq$ 90 mmHg;
- pulse $\geq$ 100 / $\geq$ 60 beats per minute.

Assessment of a patient with DKA

As previously mentioned, there is a need to be extra vigilant when assessing the older patient as their symptoms can be less overt.

In order to maintain patient safety and be responsive to potential life-threatening symptoms, the Resuscitation Council guidance on the ABCDE framework (2021b) should be used. This is a primary survey which is designed to enable the early recognition of potential life-threatening events and should enable timely interventions.

Refresh your memory of the symptoms that Veronica is demonstrating. Think about these symptoms in relation to what type of assessment you would perform. Consider what questions you would ask in order to undertake a safe and comprehensive assessment.

Airway – is the airway clear? If Veronica is talking, then her airway is not compromised at that time. Is she able to maintain a clear airway? Generally, in DKA, the patient's airway is not compromised. Veronica is breathing spontaneously; however, this may be a potential problem, particularly if her level of consciousness is reduced or she becomes unconscious. You may hear added sounds when breathing such as snoring or gurgling (sound of fluid at back of throat). Does she look cyanosed (a blue/grey tinge on the extremities or nose/tongue – remember that this assessment may be challenging in patients with dark skin, here they would look very pale)? If Veronica becomes unconscious, place her on her side and move her head back slightly. With any gurgling sounds, suctioning of the airway is required.

The odour from Veronica's breath smells fruity (acetone). This is from the presence of ketones.

Breathing – does Veronica look like she is struggling to breathe? Is she using her accessory muscles for breathing? These would be scalene, sternocleidomastoid, trapezius, abdominal muscles. Is she clammy/sweaty?

Count the respiratory rate for one full minute – is it above 25 breaths per minute? What is the pattern of her breathing? Is her breathing shallow or deep? In DKA, the patient compensates for this acidosis by deep, rapid and laboured breathing, looks like a 'deep sighing' motion known as Kussmaul breathing.

What is the pulse oximetry recording? Do remember that if the patient has a low blood pressure, the results are more likely to be inaccurate (due to poor perfusion of the finger tips).

Veronica is showing signs of Kussmaul breathing, which is caused by her low pH level. Kussmaul breathing is the body's attempt to 'blow off' carbon dioxide and compensate for acidosis.

Circulation – Veronica has a low pressure due to hypovolaemia (low blood volume).

Is her pulse weak and thready? You will need to count the pulse for one full minute, noting the rate, rhythm and strength of pulse volume. Patients with DKA may present with a weak, thready pulse. Also, count her capillary refill time (CRT). It is likely that Veronica's CRT is delayed (greater than 2 seconds). Her skin may also be cool to touch and her finger tips look pale/bluish, indicating peripheral cyanosis due to hypovolaemia.

Noting the rhythm of the pulse is also important as she may have low potassium levels causing cardiac arrhythmias to be present and the rhythm may be irregular. In the presence of arrhythmias or an irregular rhythm, an ECG should be taken, and cardiac monitoring should be considered.

Due to the dehydration, Veronica's skin is dry and her tongue is furred. There will also be a reduction in her urine output ($\leq$ 0.5 ml/k/h). Careful monitoring of her fluid intake and output is required, noting the overall balance (difference between intake and output). With DKA the patient will show a gross negative balance (more fluid output than intake).

Disability – some patients may have a lowering of their level of consciousness due to the dehydration and in severe cases be unconscious. Assess using ACPUV (Alert, confusion, responds to voice, responds to pain, unresponsive). As Veronica was fully alert, an assessment using the Glasgow Coma Scale is necessary.

Exposure – Veronica's urine should be tested for glycose and ketone levels. Bloods will also be tested for the same (capillary glucose/ketones). Whilst as an NA you will not be expected to perform these tasks (this is for the RN), you are expected to understand why this is being done.

Glycosuria and hyperglycaemia create a favourable medium for the growth of yeast organisms; consequently the patient may complain of pruritis (itching), particularly around the genitalia. So, this may be a symptom that Veronica complains of.

Also assess to see whether there are any signs of abdominal pain? If so, where is the location? How is the pain described? What is the pain intensity?

Veronica's temperature should also be monitored, particularly as she has had a fever for two days and is complaining of a sore throat.

Activity 6.5   Critical thinking

From the previous section of assessment and noting her symptoms:

- What would you consider to be Veronica's priorities in terms of care?
- Identify the management (nursing and medical interventions) for Veronica for the next six hours. Include the rationale for your answers.

An outline answer is provided at the end of this chapter.

Management of a patient with DKA

Veronica has presented with being semiconscious, hypotension and metabolic acidosis. The first 24 hours are the most critical and require very close monitoring by nurses and medical staff. Managing the patient with DKA may present a challenging situation. Initial hourly monitoring is required until the patient's condition becomes stable or improves.

The aims of treatment are to:

- decrease serum glucose;
- correct dehydration;
- correct metabolic acidosis;
- identify precipitating causes.

(JBDS, 2021)

The Joint British Diabetes Societies Framework (JBDS, 2021) for DKA provides national guidance in the management of DKA. Local protocols exist in Trusts and you are encouraged to become familiar with these. In order for treatment to prove successful the underlying cause should wherever possible be treated. Possible causes have been discussed earlier in this chapter. In the case of Veronica, as she had a history of fever and sore throat, she may have suffered from a throat infection.

The following discussions will use the framework of JBDS (2021). This framework reflects the priorities that are considered a requirement for patient management at the time of writing: Fluid replacement, insulin replacement, bedside monitoring, correcting metabolic acidosis and higher levels of care requirement. We will now explore each part of the framework in turn.

1. Fluid replacement

The main aims of fluid replacement are:

- restoration of circulatory blood volume and correct hypotension;
- clearance of ketones;
- correction of electrolyte imbalance.

(JDBS, 2021)

Fluid replacement should take account of the patient's age, degree of dehydration and issues such as history of cardiac disease. If the patient is elderly or has a history of cardiac disease, kidney failure, pregnancy, young people 18–25 (this age group is considered at high risk of developing cerebral oedema) or other serious comorbidities, the rate of fluid replacement has to be slower, otherwise there is a risk of induced heart failure caused by fluid overload.

JBDS (2021) guidelines suggest 0.9 per cent sodium chloride (normal saline) is the fluid of choice via a large bore cannula. This will also address cellular dehydration (not intravascular) as this fluid is able to enter the cells (colloids are too thick in consistency to achieve this). A colloid is a solution of large organic molecules, e.g. gelatinous solution that maintains a high osmotic pressure in the blood. A crystalloid is a solution of small molecules in water, e.g. salt. (NICE 2017b). Crystalloids are given via rapid infusion in order to restore renal blood flow and correct hypotension. The rate of infusion is titrated against the systolic blood pressure. Goals for systolic blood pressure should be given by the diabetic/medical teams.

Initial fluid replacement for a patient with systolic B/P below 90mmHg is recommended 0.9 per cent sodium chloride solution over 10–15 minutes. If systolic N/P is greater than 90 mmHg then 1 L 0.9 per cent sodium chloride over 60 minutes.

Table 6.1 represents the guidelines for fluid replacement from JBDS over the first 6 hours. You are encouraged to read the guidelines for the remaining time frames (6–24 hours).

Suggested fluid replacement for adult with no comorbidities (70kg) systolic B/P 90mmHG and above (JBDS, 2021).

Table 6.1 Fluid replacement

Fluid	Volume
0.9% sodium chloride 1L	1000ml over 1st hour
0.9% sodium chloride 1L with potassium chloride	1000ml over next 2 hours
0.9% sodium chloride 1L with potassium chloride	1000ml over next 3 hours
0.9% sodium chloride 1L with potassium chloride	1000ml over next 4 hours
0.9% sodium chloride 1L with potassium chloride	1000ml over next 5 hours
0.9% sodium chloride 1L with potassium chloride	1000ml over next 6 hours

The patient's fluid status should be reassessed by the medical team at 12 hours.

Very close attention should be paid to the monitoring of the patients (particularly the elderly and those with cardiac problems) as an infusion of too much fluid will lead to the patient having fluid overload. Signs of fluid overload include swelling of feet, hands, legs, high blood pressure, shortness of breath, expectorating clear frothy sputum.

Meticulous monitoring of vital signs such as blood pressure, pulse (rhythm, rate and depth), respiratory (rate, rhythm and depth). As previously discussed, ECG monitoring (via a cardiac monitor) should also be observed for arrhythmias associated with initial hyperkalemia; this would be demonstrated by changes to the PQRST complex. Potassium analysis (via venous blood sample) should be conducted at regular intervals for hyperkalemia and hypokalemia, as these conditions can have potentially fatal consequences (life-threatening arrhythmias). The more complex observations would be the role of the first level registered nurse (RN).

Close examination of the patient's fluid balance is a necessity to assess the level of impaired renal function, particularly in older patients or those who are physiologically unstable. Fluid balance charts should be completed on an hourly basis.

Insulin administration shifts potassium from the extracellular to the intracellular space as glucose enters the cell and restarts the membrane sodium–potassium pump. Serum potassium can fall further, thus patients are at risk of cardiac arrythmia and cardiac arrest. Regular laboratory monitoring of potassium should be performed with potassium replacement therapy when indicated.

Repletion of potassium should begin before insulin infusion if the serum potassium remains above 5.5 mmol/ (JBDS, 2021). The use of insulin will further decrease extracellular potassium levels (JBDS, 2021). This is because insulin shifts potassium from the extracellular to the intracellular space as glucose enters the cell and restarts the sodium–potassium pump.

2.   Insulin replacement

The use of insulin in the treatment of DKA is to:

- supress ketogenesis;
- reduce blood glucose;
- correct electrolyte disturbance.

(JDBS, 2021)

An intravenous infusion using a fixed scale insulin regime (capillary blood is tested at appropriate intervals and the intravenous infusion of insulin adjusted according to blood glucose levels). The type of insulin prescribed is a clinical decision by the doctor based on the patient's normal insulin therapy regime. The infusion is calculated on 0.1 unit/kilogram body weight/hr (JDBS 2021).

Once the blood glucose is less than 14 mmol/l, then 10 per cent dextrose infusion should be given and consideration to reducing the intravenous insulin infusion to 0.05 units/kg/hr. This is to prevent the onset of hypoglycaemia.

Intravenous infusions of insulin should not be stopped abruptly as the patient can become totally insulin deficient within ten minutes (causing an increase of glucose in the blood). The infusion dosage should be reduced on an hourly basis. Despite normal blood glucose levels, the infusion should not be stopped until the urine is free of ketones. Once the blood ketones are less than 0.6 mmol/l and venous pH greater than 7.3 and the patient is eating, subcutaneous insulin can be commenced. Again, the type of insulin is dependent upon the patient's normal regime. Hypoglycaemia is one complication that should be avoided through careful monitoring.

3.   Bedside monitoring

The checking of blood ketone measurements is considered to be best practice in monitoring the patient's response to treatment. This is a process via a ketone meter, with results in minutes. It is a nursing task that requires further training at Trust level. Capillary blood glucose levels should also be closely monitored, initially on an hourly basis until the patient's condition improves. The use of laboratory measurements will be required when the results are 'out of range' of the meters. Normal values for blood ketones are lower than 0.6 mmol/L (NHS, 2021a).

Regular monitoring of venous blood gas (for bicarbonate and pH levels). This is another task that will be performed by the RN or doctor.

4. Correcting metabolic acidosis

If the patient's condition is severe enough to develop metabolic acidosis, they are likely to be transferred to higher levels of care. It is outside of the remit of this book to discuss this area. If you would like to gain knowledge in this area, please consult the JDBS (2021) guidelines on DKA.

5. Higher levels of care requirement

Signs of deterioration/criteria for admission to higher levels of care (e.g. high dependency unit). These include:

- high risk patients (identified earlier);
- severe DKA – venous Ph below 7.1;
- hypokalaemia (below 3.5 mmol/l);
- GCS less than 12;
- oxygen saturation below 92% (on room air);
- systolic B/P less than 90mmHg;
- pulse greater than 100 or less than 60 bpm;
- central venous pressure (CVP) monitoring.

(JBDS 2021)

Health promotion

In many instances, the occurrence of DKA is preventable (mainly through patient education), and so the role of the nurse as a health educator/promoter is essential.

Once the priorities of management and care have been addressed for Veronica, consideration should then be given to health promotion. The focus here is on prevention of further episodes. The importance of preventing disease as far as possible in relation to causative factors of DKA, for example, common cold, infection etc. should be emphasised. Tips should also be given to Veronica on how to manage any stress/stressful situations that she finds herself experiencing. Food and nutrition management should be revisited and the importance of continuing with her insulin therapy when ill (even when experiencing nausea and vomiting from other illness) should be explained. Veronica may need to be re-educated regarding the need to monitor her blood glucose regularly and how to do this accurately.

Some patients, including Veronica, may find it extremely difficult to implement the recommendations by healthcare professionals in relation to modifying diet: complying with self-monitoring; taking of medication; adapting personal lifestyle habits and returning for follow-up. Healthcare professionals should work with patients to identify and agree a plan of action. Recommended techniques for patient education and counselling provide factual information and motivational encouragement (needed for meaningful change) should be adopted.

Chapter summary

This particular chapter has referred to the JBDS (2021), which provide current standards and clinical guidance for the management of DKA at the time of writing. The physiology of normal blood glucose control has been discussed. Understanding the pathophysiology of DKA will help to gain knowledge and understanding of its symptoms. The ABCDE approach to assessment has been used based on a case study. The criteria for escalating concerns and possible transfer of patient to higher levels of care have also been included.

Activities: brief outline answers

Activity 6.2 Critical thinking

Required for normal brain, renal medulla and red blood cell functioning. Provides an energy source for their function.

Glucose is controlled by the pancreas, and the hormones involved in the control of glucose are insulin and glucagon. Insulin promotes the transportation of glucose into the cells and lowers blood glucose levels. Glucagon breaks down glucose and fat, resulting in the increase of blood glucose levels.

Intake of too much carbohydrate. Production of insulin in the pancreas.

Activity 6.3 Critical thinking

Hyperglycaemia

  high blood glucose levels;
  glycosuria (high levels of glucose in urine);
  pruritus (itching – particularly around the genitalia);
  polydipsia (increased thirst);
  polyurea (increased urine output).

Dehydration

  lowered blood pressure;
  increased pulse;
  dry skin/furred tongue;
  decreased urine output.

Electrolyte loss

  potassium – cardiac arrhythmias;
  low magnesium – cardiac arrhythmia;
  low phosphate – cardiac arrhythmias.

Ketoacidosis

  acetone smell on breath;
  Kussmaul breathing;
  ketones in blood and urine.

Activity 6.4 Critical thinking

Veronica demonstrates the following in relation to the criteria:
  pulse ≥ 100 / ≥ 60 beats per minute – pulse is 140.
  Please note that whilst the rest of her observations do not achieve the criteria they are *very* borderline. This means that her condition can deteriorate very quickly and is showing the signs of severe DKA.

correct dehydration;
reduction of high blood glucose levels;
correct metabolic acidosis;
identify precipitating causes.

Identify the management (nursing and medical interventions) for Veronica for the next six hours.

Fluid replacement following JBDS (2021) guidance. Monitor vital signs and fluid balance.
Fixed insulin infusion – monitoring of blood glucose and ketones

Further reading

British Society of Paediatric Endocrinology and Diabetes (2020). BSPED interim guideline for the **management of children and young people under the age of 18 years with diabetic ketoacidosis.** www.sort.nhs.uk/Media/Guidelines/BSPED-DKA-guideline-2020-update.pdf

This is a substantial guidance document that covers all aspects of managing children and young people with DKA. It includes diagnosis, emergency management, assessment, ongoing management and medication management. This is especially useful for NAs or student NAs working with children.

Diabetes.co.uk (2022). Diabetic Ketoacidosis (DKA). www.diabetes.co.uk/diabetes-complications/diabetic-ketoacidosis.html

This is a useful resource for patients from a major source of information for them in the United Kingdom; it is user friendly and therefore a useful initial resource for NA students.

Royal College of Nursing (2020) Education, prevention and the role of the nursing team. www.rcn.org.uk/clinical-topics/Diabetes/Education-prevention-and-the-role-of-the-nurse

This is a useful resource that provides an overview of the role of the nurse within diabetes services, focused on patient education, and also provides links to further resources.

World Health Organisation (2021) Diabetes. www.who.int/news-room/fact-sheets/detail/diabetes

This is a useful resource from the WHO providing an overview of diabetes and how the WHO is responding to the challenges on a global scale.

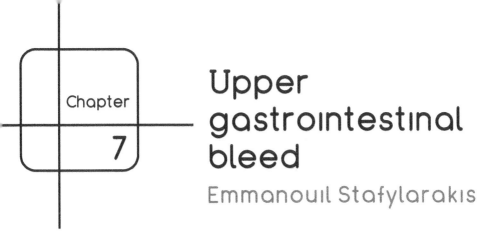

Chapter 7

Upper gastrointestinal bleed

Emmanouil Stafylarakis

(Continued)

Annexe A: Communication and relationship management skills

Nursing associates need a diverse range of communication skills and strategies to ensure that individuals, their families and carers are supported to be actively involved in their own care wherever appropriate, and that they are kept informed and well prepared.

At the point of registration, the nursing associate will be able to:

1.1:   actively listen, recognise and respond to verbal and non-verbal cues

Chapter aims

By the end of the chapter, you will be able to:

- define what is meant by the term gastro-intestinal (GI) bleeding and identify the types and associated risk factors/triggers;
- discuss basic anatomy and physiology of the upper GI system;
- explain the underpinning pathophysiology of upper GI bleeding;
- understand how to appropriately assess a patient with upper GI bleeding;
- identify the priorities of nursing care for a patient with upper GI bleeding.

Introduction

Upper gastro-intestinal (GI) bleeding is a common, often life-threatening medical emergency. The estimated annual incidence of GI bleed in the UK is 85,000 patients per year, approximately presenting every six minutes (National Confidential Enquiry into Patient Outcomes and Deaths (NCEPOD, 2015a). In the last 20 years, the mortality rate for acute upper GI bleeding has remained high in the UK, with 9,000 deaths per annum (Ahmed and Stanley, 2012). Upper GI bleeding can only be treated in a hospital setting and its severity is evaluated through risk assessment of the patient. This allows for timely escalation of care, mortality prediction and appropriate patient discharge planning. This chapter will present a case study, José, and explore the priorities of treatment and patient care, which involve an emergency endoscopy. An endoscopy means 'looking inside' and refers to any instrument used to examine the interior of a hollow organ or cavity of the body. For upper GI, it is often used interchangeably with oesophago-gastro-duodenoscopy (OGD) (NCEPOD, 2015a). José's case study will include his journey following admission to A&E, transfer to the operating theatres department for an emergency OGD for suspected upper GI bleeding, and transfer to the high dependency unit (HDU) for closer monitoring and treatment. The learning from this chapter will be useful for you as a NA student or a registered NA if you are caring for a patient with GI bleeding in a range of settings.

Case study: José, the GI patient

You are a nursing associate (NA) student undertaking a placement in the operating theatres department. Your practice supervisor has suggested you observe the multidisciplinary team (MDT) preparing to receive a patient who was admitted in the A&E department an hour ago. The patient's name is José. 80 years old. His past medical history includes atrial fibrillation (AF), hypertension and ischaemic heart disease. José takes aspirin and warfarin for his AF. He is a non-smoker, with minimal alcohol intake. On admission to A&E, José complains of black faeces, known as melaena, chest tightness and upper abdominal pain. He is anxious, with an increasing shortness of breath. José has been diagnosed for potential upper GI bleeding. In A&E, due to a rapid decrease of blood pressure and haemoglobin and increased heart rate, José was assessed to have an emergency OGD in the theatres department to be investigated or treated for the source of bleeding in the upper GI and potential need for surgery. He is communicative, and his vital signs were as follows:

- heart rate (HR): 92 beats per minute (bpm);
- blood pressure (BP): 115/75 millimetres of mercury (mmHg);
- respiratory rate (RR): 22 breaths per minute (bpm);
- saturations (SpO2): 95% on room air;
- temperature (TEMP): 36.3 °C.

Activity 7.1   Critical thinking

Using Figure 2.4 NEWS2 and Figure 2.5 NEWS2 Thresholds and triggers in Chapter 2, calculate José's NEWS2 score in A&E, and identify whether there is a clinical risk and what response should be actioned for José.

An outline answer is given at the end of the chapter.

Anatomy and physiology of the GI system

To begin to understand how to care for a patient with a GI bleed it is important to understand the anatomy and physiology of the GI system and blood supply to the liver (portal circulation, see Figure 7.1). This section will provide a brief overview of the upper and lower parts of the digestive system and their basic functionality and emphasis will be given to the upper part due to the condition being addressed within the case study. By knowing the essential anatomy and physiology you will be able to imagine the parts of the upper GI tract; from the mouth to the ligament of Treitz, the boundary between duodenum and jejunum. This will help you to understand the upper GI bleeding presentation signs and identify the patient's needs.

The digestive system consists of the gastrointestinal tract (GI) and the axillary organs, which are the salivary glands, liver and pancreas. The GI tract consists of five layers of different types of tissue which are, from the innermost, the mucosa to the submucosa, muscularis, and up to the outermost, the serosa, which is surrounded from the mesentery. Figure 7.2 outlines these components of the GI system and associated function.

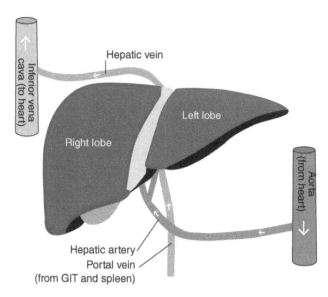

Figure 7.1 Blood supply to the liver (Cook, 2021)

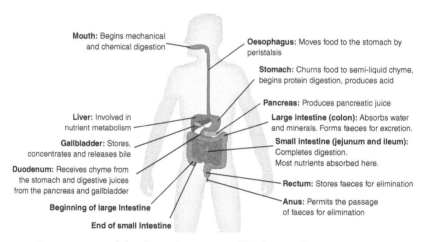

Figure 7.2 Components of the digestive system (Cook, 2021)

Activity 7.2   Reflection

Using Figure 7.1, list the function of the oesophagus, stomach, liver, pancreas, large and small intestine, gallbladder, duodenum and rectum. Doing this exercise will support your understanding of GI anatomy and physiology.

As this activity is based on your own reflection, no outline answer is provided at the end of this chapter.

Definition and types of upper GI bleeding

An upper GI bleed refers to bleeding from the oesophagus, stomach or duodenum. In this medical emergency the patient bleeds from either the oesophagus or stomach or duodenum or simultaneously from all those GI segments (see Figure 7.1 for function and location). This bleeding is caused by various factors which have been grouped, based on their origin, into variceal and non-variceal bleeding.

> Variceal describes bleeding of varices, which are formations of the anastomotic veins of the oesophagus, stomach and duodenum's outer and sub-mucosal walls, due to portal hypertension. In these formations, due to increased blood pressure, the anastomotic veins become enlarged and are more likely to burst (Cook et al., 2019; Sharma and Rameshbabu, 2012).

> Non-variceal describes bleeding of the oesophagus, stomach and duodenum's mucosa wall due to inflammatory diseases, irritation, fibrotic tissue formation, infection, medication, vasoconstriction induced ischaemia and peptic ulcers (Cook et al., 2019).

A GI bleed is approximately 8 to 9 times more likely to be non-variceal than variceal (Alzoubaidi et al., 2019). Non-variceal upper GI bleeding is more frequent in the elderly population than in younger people due to the use of non-steroidal anti-inflammatory drugs (NSAIDs) and aspirin, potential infection with Helicobacter pylori (H. pylori), comorbidities and age. Some older adults use one or more antiplatelet agents and NSAIDs to prevent blood thrombosis, reduce the risks of cardiovascular and/or cerebrovascular episodes and to treat rheumatological conditions. H. pylori infection has been recognised as a factor that can cause peptic ulcer disease and, when combined with the use of NSAIDs, can result in peptic ulcer bleeding (Ahmed and Stanley, 2012).

The signs of suspected upper GI bleeding are haematemesis (vomiting of blood), coffee-ground vomiting, melaena or unexplained fall in haemoglobin. This is a frightening experience for the patient, involving fear of death and stress, and it needs an interdisciplinary team approach to provide care in a timely manner. The timing of the relevant care is crucial to patient survival, as upper GI bleeding may lead to hypovolaemic shock and death.

Associated risk factors for upper GI bleeding

The risk factors for upper GI bleeding are related to the nature of the bleeding, variceal or no-variceal, patient demographics, gender and age, lifestyle, emotional status, bacterial infection, medications, aortoenteric fistulas, post-surgical bleeds, foreign body ingestion and iatrogenically, as well as the patient's past medical history of diseases, malignant tumours and comorbidities (Cook et al., 2019; Sharma and Rameshbabu, 2012; Ahmed and Stanley, 2012; DiGregorio and Alvey, 2021).

Pathophysiology of upper GI bleed

An upper GI bleeding is caused by two general pathophysiological pathways based on the origin of the bleeding, variceal or non-variceal.

Variceal bleeding occurs where enlarged varices of the anastomotic veins, usually the lower part of the oesophagus and stomach and, rarely, the duodenum (see Figure 7.1), are burst due to the portal hypertension. The portal hypertension regards the increased blood pressure in the portal vein (see Figure 7.2) due to major inflammatory conditions, mainly thrombosis or cirrhosis of the liver where the blood flow is impeded. The varices in the lower part of the oesophagus and stomach are bigger than those of the duodenum. The formation of varices in the anastomotic veins of the upper GI tract appear in the outermost layer, the serosa, and in the submucosa wall. In the submucosa wall the varices or their stigmata of previous bleeding can be visible through an OGD endoscopy (Cook et al., 2019; Sharma and Rameshbabu, 2012; Ahmed and Stanley, 2012).

Non-variceal bleeding varies according to the location, the origin of the risk or triggering factors. In the oesophagus, an increase in the intra-abdominal pressure, for example due to pregnancy, constipation and obesity or low levels of the hormone gastrin or presence of hiatus hernia, can cause gastro-oesophageal reflux.

Gastro-oesophageal reflux is a disease that is caused by persistent regurgitation of gastric acid into the oesophagus. The gastric acid is extremely acidic and therefore irritating, and causes inflammation and painful ulceration. In these conditions, the blood vessels of the oesophagus are eroded and bleed.

'Barrett's oesophagus' is a long-lasting gastro-oesophageal reflux that is associated with a pre-malignant condition and sometimes accompanied by hiatus hernia. Adenocarcinoma can develop from Barrett's oesophagus. Other tumours, such as a squamous cell carcinoma in the lower part of the oesophagus (see Figure 7.2), begin as an ulcer that spreads round the circumference, causing stricture and resulting in dysphagia. In this condition prognosis can be poor. The risk factors for the development of the squamous cell carcinoma are alcohol intake and cigarette smoking and other factors related to unhealthy lifestyle.

Gastritis is inflammation of the stomach, which can be acute or chronic. Acute gastritis is caused by irritant drugs and alcohol. The most common irritants are the non-steroidal anti-inflammatory drugs (NSAIDs) and aspirin (Cook et al., 2019). In the elderly, an acute upper GI bleeding related to acute gastritis can be due to the combination of NSAIDs and/or chronic gastritis induced by the H.pylori (Ahmed and Stanley, 2012). Bleeding occurs due to erosions of the gastric mucosa and chronic gastritis is commonly associated with peptic ulcer disease.

Acute gastritis can develop due to severe stress, major surgery, shock and burns, as well as severe emotional disturbance, which can lead to acute peptic ulcers in the stomach, leading to bleeding. A possible life-threatening bleeding as a complication of peptic ulcers occurs when a major artery is eroded, causing hypovolaemic shock, haematemesis and/or melaena (Cook et al., 2019).

Assessing the acutely ill upper GI bleeding patient

Having identified a patient at risk of upper GI bleeding, the next step is to carry out a full comprehensive patient assessment, utilising the ABCDE (airway, breathing, circulation, disability, exposure) approach (RCUK, 2021b) and signs of blood (Table 7.1, 7.2). This is a systematic structure that is implemented for José's vital assessment status prior to his transfer to the operating department.

Table 7.1   ABCDE assessment of José

First steps	• personal safety
	• ask José how he is
Airway	• José has not shown signs of airway obstruction and is maintaining his own airway in A&E
Breathing	• signs of increasing shortness of breath
	• respiratory rate (RR): 24 bpm
	• saturations (SpO2): 94% on room air
	• listen to José's breath sounds, and check if equal and bilateral rise and fall of the chest wall
	• percuss and auscultate José's chest (if trained to do so)
Circulation	• look at the colour of José's hands and fingers
	• measure José's capillary refill time
	• assess the state of José's veins and urine output status
	• observe for further black faeces (melena) through stool chart
	• heart rate (HR): 95 bpm
	• blood pressure (BP): 110/60 mmHg
	• temperature (TEMP): 36.1°C
	• ascertain IV access status
	• complete a 12-lead ECG
	• take blood from the cannula for routine haematological, biochemical, coagulation investigations and cross-matching
Disability	• Glasgow Coma Scale (GCS) 15/15, alert
	• examine José's pupil size and measure blood glucose level
Exposure	• examine the patient properly from head to toe
	• respect the patient's dignity and minimise heat loss

Table 7.2   Regular observations for signs of blood in José's faeces or vomit

Observe if occurs	• blood existence in vomit and document time and blood volume
	• blood in faeces using a stool chart
Stool chart	• label the stool chart with the patient's hospital ID
	• add date
	• document regularly:
	○ time
	○ colour
	○ consistency (Use Bristol stool Chart)
	○ blood (yes or no)
	○ mucous (yes or no)
	○ amount

By assessing signs of a GI bleed in stools and vomit, you record blood loss and monitor frequency of bleeding. A fall in blood pressure and urine output which cause an increase in heart rate may indicate a significant blood loss. After this comprehensive assessment you report your findings based on the local policy. This is explored in Activity 7.3 using NEWS scores which were discussed in Chapter 2.

Activity 7.3   Critical thinking

Using Figure 2.4 NEWS2, and Figure 2.5 NEWS2 Thresholds and triggers in Chapter 2, calculate José's NEWS2 score prior to transfer to the operating theatres, and identify whether there is a clinical risk and what response should be actioned for José. Reflect on any difference with Activity 7.1.

An outline answer is given at the end of the chapter.

The WHO surgical safety checklist

Clinical errors cause significant morbidity, mortality and increased cost across the NHS and there is increasing evidence that use of checklists can reduce errors and improve patient survivor and well-being (Mason et al., 2018).

The World Health Organization (WHO, 2018) produced and recommended the basic layout of a surgical safety checklist in 2009 and provided a performance update in 2018 which has been adapted by many hospitals across the world and modified based on the local needs (Weiser and Haynes, 2018). It provides an opportunity for the MDT to check and share vital information for patient safety before a procedure starts. For endoscopic and surgical procedures, this information is documented on one form during patient preparation, before procedure and after procedure times. The local endoscopy safety checklist has been designed and used to ensure the patient is adequately prepared for endoscopy. Also, it is a tool for the handover between ward and endoscopy nursing teams or operating theatres and recovery unit depending on where the endoscopy procedure took place. This will be explored in the developing case study below.

Case study: José (continued)

To investigate the type of upper GI bleeding and determine treatment, José is transferred to the operating department for an OGD. There is a considerable risk of a major haemorrhage, thus the operating theatre staff should be aware of the need for open surgery to address the bleeding if this does occur. This is a decision made by the medical team based on the patient's high risk status due to past medical history and comorbidities, and staff skills as well as availability of relevant equipment. José is informed and consent is obtained for general anaesthesia, which includes endotracheal intubation. The anaesthetist monitors the haemodynamic status of the patient and manages fluid balance, and blood is made available in case it is needed. You and the

(Continued)

(Continued)

rest of the nursing team pay attention to safe manual handling, preparation of equipment for the procedure, communication with José, care plan and documentation. The theatre staff who are looking after José intraoperatively must be aware of the major haemorrhage protocol and how to activate it in case José has a major haemorrhage during the OGD procedure.

Hunt et al. (2015) provide some key recommendations for management of a patient such as José with a major haemorrhage. These include that hospitals must have local major haemorrhage protocols which reference different clinical areas, and that all key staff have access to this and are familiar with it. Additionally medical and nursing staff should be trained in the recognition of major blood loss at early stages, and when to activate the local policy for management of this (Hunt et al., 2015).

Major haemorrhage management guideline

In order to understand the risk of blood loss for a patient under GI bleed and the possibility that bleeding will develop into a major haemorrhage, a practical guideline for the management of major haemorrhage in the local clinical settings is recommended by Hunt et al. (2015) as shown in Figure 7.3.

Having reviewed this useful guidance, it is now helpful to consider how this is applied in your own place of work in the following activity.

Activity 7.4   Critical thinking

Explore in your clinical setting what major haemorrhage protocol is in effect and compare the steps against the practical guideline of Figure 7.3. Reflect on the similarities and differences as well as considering your role as a member of the multidisciplinary team in the application of such a protocol.

As this activity is based on your own experience, no outline answer is provided at the end of the chapter.

Treatment options for upper GI bleed

The therapeutic interventions are divided into those for **non-variceal bleeding** and those for **variceal bleeding**, as follows:

Non-variceal bleeding therapeutic interventions

- injection – of adrenaline to cause vein vasoconstriction in the peptic ulcers area, reducing re-bleeding rate (Kahi et al., 2005);

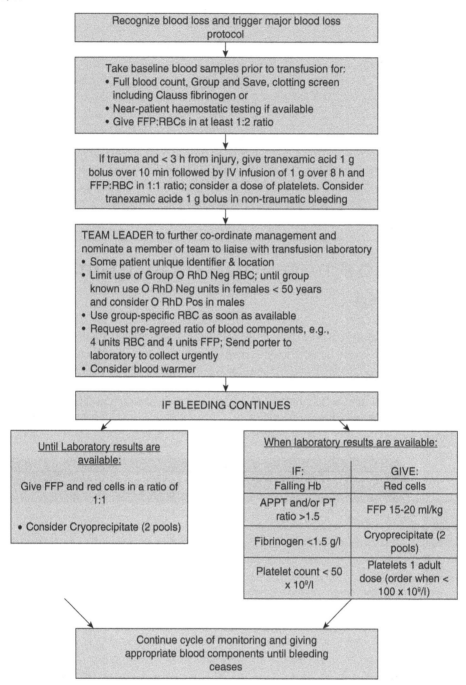

Figure 7.3 A practical guideline for the haematological management of major haemorrhage (Hunt et al., 2015)

- thermal treatment – to seal the vein erosions through heating (NICE, 2016a);
- mechanical treatment – by compressing the veins on the bleeding lesions through stainless steel clips (NICE, 2016a);
- hemospray – which consists of a haemostatic powder that is spread over the vessel lesions and facilitates the clotting process by stopping the bleeding (Tang et al., 2019).

Variceal bleeding therapeutic interventions

- variceal bleeding ligation – small rubber band surrounding the varix, causes transfixion and stops bleeding (NICE 2016);
- glue injection – into bleeding vessels by hardening and occluding the varix to stop bleeding (Castellanos et al., 2012);
- balloon tamponade – through a Sengstaken–Blakemore tube insertion from the mouth to the stomach. The tube carries a balloon across its length and by inflation with sterile liquid the balloon tamponades, i.e. pressures the bled varices to stop bleeding to the area of oesophagus or stomach or both (Tripathi et al., 2015);
- oesophageal stenting – an alternative to balloon tamponade, this is a self-expanding metal tube applying pressure to the varices to stop bleeding (McCarty and Njei, 2016);

We will now review these treatment options by returning to our case study, José.

Case study: José (continued)

Intra-operatively, José was treated for peptic ulcers, which was the main cause of the bleeding. Post-operatively, he recovered in the Post-Anaesthesia Care Unit (PACU) for a short period of time and then was transferred to the HDU. In HDU, his vital signs were as follows:

- heart rate (HR): 70 beats per minute (bpm);
- blood pressure (BP): 135/80 millimetres of mercury (mmHg);
- respiratory rate (RR): 18 breaths per minute (bpm);
- saturations (SpO2): 97% (provided with oxygen 2 Litres per minute);
- temperature (TEMP): 36.5 °C.

José is now therefore in the post-operative phase of his care and, as can be seen, his clinical observations are within normal parameters.

Priorities of care for patient care post-endoscopy for upper GI bleed

The priorities of care post-endoscopy are the following:

- implement a comprehensive ABCDE assessment in the recommended frequency stated in the post-endoscopy instructions on the patient notes;
- escalate care immediately, if a fall in BP of more than 20mmHg is observed, or an increase in HR of more than 20 bpm, based on the local policy;
- regularly assess signs of blood in faeces and/or vomit and report your findings to a physician;
- regularly assess urine output based on the patient's weight using the minimum normal rate of 0.5ml/Kg/hour to document type of diuresis and record amounts of fluid intake for fluid balance planning.

Within the next activity these priorities of care will be reviewed in relation to José to enhance your application of this knowledge.

Activity 7.5   Critical thinking

Using Figure 2.4 NEWS2 and Figure 2.5 NEWS2 Thresholds and triggers in Chapter 2, calculate José's NEWS2 score in HDU, and identify whether there is a clinical risk and what response should be actioned for José. Observe the trends in this and previous observations from Activities 7.1 and 7.3 regarding the vital signs, RR, SpO2, BP and HR. Reflect on José's homeostatic mechanisms to compensate hypovolaemia (low blood volume) due to bleeding.

An outline answer is given at the end of the chapter.

Chapter summary

This chapter has discussed the care of a patient with upper GI bleeding based on current evidence. The case study of José is used as an example to explore the management of this condition and care delivery. José is admitted to A&E but transferred to the operating theatres for an urgent procedure to diagnose and treat his suspected upper GI bleed. NA students and NAs can provide a vital role in caring for patients such as José, using knowledge of relevant anatomy, physiology, pathophysiology and patient deterioration monitoring skills as reviewed within this chapter. An urgent endoscopy and transfer from A&E to the operating department is a frightening experience for the patient. A patient's comprehensive ABCDE assessment and signs of blood have been explored as priorities of care. Care of patients before, during and after emergency OGD has been discussed. The chapter has included activities to encourage application of the concepts explored and encourage deeper thinking, with further reading and websites provided.

Activities: brief outline answers

Activity 7.1 Critical thinking

NEWS2 = 4. Based on this NEWS2, the clinical risk is low. However, you should consider that in A&E José can suddenly deteriorate. So, the prespecified clinical response by the RCP (2017) must be considered in the context of effective communication, keeping the registered nurse informed and continuously assessing the patient. Namely, in A&E and other critical care settings the vital signs are affected by other risk factors for the patient, e.g. active bleeding, which limit the time for rescuing. Thus, the frequency of monitoring is dependent on those factors.

Activity 7.3 Critical thinking

NEWS2 = 5. Based on this NEWS2, the clinical risk is medium, and José has deteriorated in a very short time during his A&E stay. You have already informed the registered nurse. The medical team is around José, including anaesthetists who are assessing the patient for transferring to the operating theatres along with portal monitoring facilities. The change, which is observed as a calculation outcome in the NEWS2, is due to the rapid drop in the systolic blood pressure.

Activity 7.5 Critical thinking

NEWS2 = 2. Based on this NEWS2, the clinical risk is low. However, you should consider that in the HDU, José can suddenly deteriorate due to re-bleeding with consequent blood loss. So, the prespecified clinical response by the RCP (2017) must be considered in the context of effective communication, keeping the registered nurse informed and continuously assessing the patient. Namely, in HDU and other critical care settings the vital signs are affected by other risk factors for the patient, e.g. organ decline due to hypovolaemia and hence hypoxia, which limit the time for rescuing. Thus, the frequency of monitoring is dependent on those factors. José's active bleeding in A&E, which caused his sudden deterioration, manifested a fall in BP of which the systolic blood pressure (SBP) was used for the calculation in those NEWS2 totals, i.e. on José's arrival in A&E and pre-operatively. The fall in the diastolic blood pressure from 75 to 60 mmHg can indicate arterial vasodilation. Due to José's blood loss and consequent hypovolaemia, cardiac output is reduced. Thus, you can consider signs of reduced urine output below the minimum normal rate 0.5ml/Kg/hour (Shepherd, 2011, page 15) or poor organ perfusion causing chest pain. Fluid balance approach by the MDT facilitated José's body homeostatic mechanisms to compensate hypovolaemia, reducing RR and increasing SpO2, as more blood volume can transfer more oxygen to the tissues, increasing blood pressure and decreasing HR as an indication of an increased cardiac output.

Further reading

Chapman, W., Siau, K., Thomas, F., Ernest, S., Begum, S., Iqbal, T. and Bhala, N. (2019) Acute upper gastrointestinal bleeding: a guide for nurses. British Journal of Nursing (Mark Allen Publishing), 28(1): 53–59.

This article outlines the latest evidence-based care for patients with acute upper GI bleeding. It aims to help gastroenterology and general medical ward nurses and nursing associates plan nursing interventions and understand the diagnostic treatment options available.

Stanley, A.J. and Laine, L. (2019) Management of acute upper gastrointestinal bleeding. British Medical Journal (Clinical research ed.), 364: l536.

This article involves medicine, baseline and alternative diagnostic and therapeutic procedures as an overview about upper GI bleeding. The information included in this article familiarises endoscopy nurses and nursing associates with the medical needs of the patient in order to communicate effectively with the MDT, the patient and relatives, as well as preparing equipment for the interventional procedures.

Weledji, E.P. (2020) Acute upper gastrointestinal bleeding: a review. *Surgery in Practice and Science*, 1: 100004.

This article involves medicine and emergency surgery related to upper GI bleeding, highlighting the need for effective MDT and departmental communication. The information included in this article familiarises endoscopy and theatre nurses as well as nursing associates with the medical and emergency surgery needs of the patient in order to communicate effectively with the MDT, the patient and relatives, as well as preparing equipment for the interventional procedures and potential surgery.

Useful websites

www.ncepod.org.uk/2015gih.html

The National Confidential Enquiry into Patient Outcome and Death: Gastrointestinal Haemorrhage: Time to Get Control?

www.resus.org.uk/

Resuscitation Council UK

www.rcplondon.ac.uk/projects/outputs/national-early-warning-score-news-2

National Early Warning Score (NEWS) 2

www.glasgowcomascale.org/

Glasgow Coma Scale

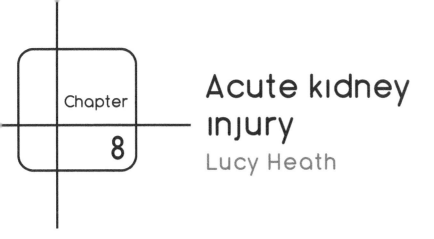

Chapter 8

Acute kidney injury

Lucy Heath

NMC STANDARDS OF PROFICIENCY FOR NURSING ASSOCIATES

This chapter will address the following platforms and proficiencies:

Platform 2: Promoting health and preventing ill health

At the point of registration the nursing associate will be able to:

2.1   understand and apply the aims and principles of health promotion, protection and improvement and the prevention of ill health when engaging with people

2.2   promote preventive health behaviours and provide information to support people to make informed choices to improve their mental, physical and behavioural health and well-being

Platform 3: Provide and monitor care

At the point of registration, the nursing associate will be able to:

3.2   demonstrate and apply knowledge of body systems and homeostasis, human anatomy and physiology, biology, genomics, pharmacology, social and behavioural sciences when delivering care

3.3   recognise and apply knowledge of commonly encountered mental, physical, behavioural and cognitive health conditions when delivering care

3.4   demonstrate the knowledge, communication and relationship management skills required to provide people, families and carers with accurate information that meets their needs before, during and after a range of interventions

3.6   demonstrate the knowledge, skills and ability to perform a range of nursing procedures and manage devices, to meet people's need for safe, effective and person-centred care

Chapter aims

By the end of this chapter you will be able to:

- define what is meant by the term 'acute kidney injury' and presenting symptoms;
- discuss basic anatomy and physiology of a normal renal system;
- explain the underpinning pathophysiology of acute kidney injury;
- understand how to assess a patient with an acute kidney injury;
- discuss the priorities of care for a patient with an acute kidney injury;
- understand how to manage a patient with an acute kidney injury, including pharmacology;
- discuss health promotion related to the prevention of a patient developing an acute kidney injury.

Introduction

Within the hospital setting, an acute kidney injury (AKI), previously known as acute renal failure, is a common condition among in-patients, with around 10–20 per cent acquiring the condition during their admission (Nagalingam, 2019). An AKI can range from a slight impairment to severe deterioration of function, but is a rapid deterioration that can be life threatening (Hulse and Davies, 2015). An AKI is a reversible condition with patients being able to make a complete recovery with no complications. Although reversible, this depends on the level of damage that has occurred and whether timely management and treatment has been received (Nagalingam, 2019). It is important to consider that an AKI is often accompanied by other medical conditions, which can prevent a patient from recovering as easily as this. AKI has been previously referred to as acute renal failure, so you may notice this term in older texts and when in practice.

This chapter will discuss the role of the nursing associate (NA) within the care of a patient with AKI; this will focus on a case study.

Case study: Dilys, the AKI patient

Dilys is a 77-year-old female attending A&E with shortness of breath, oedema and oliguria. Vital signs were recorded:

- heart rate: 127 beats per minute (BPM);
- blood pressure: 178/102 millimetres of mercury (mmHg);
- respiration rate: 28 breaths per minute;
- saturations (SpO2): 96%;
- temperature: 36.7 °C;
- conscious level using ACVPU (alert, confusion, voice, pain, unresponsive) scale: alert.

Bloods were taken on admission, including venous blood gas (VBG), which was available within a few minutes. VBG demonstrated hyperkalemia (6.5 millimoles per litre) and acidosis (pH 7.26). An electrocardiogram (ECG) was recorded, which was displaying atrial fibrillation (AF), which was a previously known diagnosis. Dilys was placed on a cardiac monitor due to the hyperkalemia for ongoing monitoring.

(Continued)

(Continued)

Blood results demonstrate hyperkalemia, raised urea and creatinine and a lowered estimated glomerular filtration rate (eGFR). Dilys usually takes furosemide and ramipril as she has congestive cardiac failure (CCF) and hypertension and she takes rivaroxiban for AF. She advised nursing staff that she did not drink much in the day as she needs to pass urine regularly and is struggling with her mobility. She also has arthritis so is prescribed naproxen from her GP for the pain. Dilys is diagnosed with an AKI and worsening CCF. She is admitted onto a medical ward for management.

This case study of Dilys will be referred to throughout the chapter when addressing pathophysiology, assessment and management of AKI.

Defining acute kidney injury

An AKI can be described as rapidly decreased renal function, which in turn results in an inability to maintain fluid and electrolyte balance. It is a suddenly occurring condition identified by a raise in creatinine compared to a previous baseline figure (Hulse and Davies, 2015). The severity can be mild, moderate or severe, although even a mild AKI can result in permanent kidney damage and reduction in kidney function (Tait and Hansen, 2016). An AKI significantly increases both mortality and morbidity of patients (Woodrow, 2015). Kanagasundaram et al. (2019) advise that preventative measures should be put in place for high risk groups rather than waiting for an AKI to develop and be treated.

High risk groups for developing an AKI are listed below:

- chronic kidney disease (adults with an estimated glomerular filtration rate [eGFR] less than 60 ml/min/1.73 m 2 are at particular risk);
- heart failure;
- liver disease;
- diabetes;
- history of acute kidney injury;
- oliguria (urine output less than 0.5 ml/kg/hour);
- neurological or cognitive impairment or disability, which may mean limited access to fluids because of reliance on a carer;
- hypovolaemia;
- use of drugs that can cause or exacerbate kidney injury (such as non-steroidal anti-inflammatory drugs (NSAIDs), aminoglycosides, angiotensin-converting enzyme (ACE) inhibitors, angiotensin II receptor antagonists (ARBs) and diuretics) within the past week, especially if hypovolaemic;
- use of iodine-based contrast media within the past week;
- symptoms or history of urological obstruction, or conditions that may lead to obstruction;
- sepsis;
- deteriorating early warning scores;
- age 65 years or over.

(NICE, 2019b)

It is helpful to review these pre-existing conditions in relation to Dilys; this is considered in the following activity.

Activity 8.1   Critical thinking

What pre-existing conditions would make Dilys at high risk of developing an AKI?
An outline answer is provided at the end of this chapter.

Symptoms of AKI

The main symptoms presented by Dilys of AKI are oliguria, fluid retention, nausea, shortness of breath, confusion, drowsiness, oedema and dehydration. Rapid onset is expected. As an AKI is often secondary to another condition, it can be challenging to link the symptoms to an AKI rather than another condition (Hulse and Davies, 2015). In the case study, Dilys was admitted with shortness of breath, but this is also a symptom of heart failure, which is another diagnosis she has.

An increase in creatinine is an early indicator of AKI, as well as urine output of less than 0.5mls/kg. Oliguria is usually caused by a lack of blood flow to the kidneys, although a post renal cause will need to be excluded. Completion of a bladder scan will confirm whether any urine is reaching the bladder. Should the bladder be full and the patient in urinary retention, catheterisation is necessary. Depending on the cause of the retention, a supra pubic catheter may need to be inserted by a specialist. This would be due to a urethral blockage, such as an enlarged prostate, or renal calculi obstructing the urethra, preventing a catheter passing through to the bladder.

Mortality from AKI

Mortality from AKI is documented as between 25 and 30 per cent (Nagalingam, 2019) and 50 per cent (Jones and Steggall, 2020). The condition mostly affects elderly individuals with comorbidities, hence the high rate of mortality identified within the literature. Patients will rarely present with an AKI alone. Usually it is an incidental finding on completing blood tests and monitoring urine output. In the case study, Dilys attended A&E as she was symptomatic of worsening heart failure, but an AKI was incidentally found through blood tests and oliguria.

Chronic kidney disease and AKI

AKI is not to be confused with chronic kidney disease (CKD) which is a long-term condition rather than acute illness. However, left untreated, an AKI can deteriorate into CKD (Hulse and Davies, 2015). Individuals who have had an AKI are at higher risk of developing CKD in the future.

Basic anatomy and physiology of the renal system

It is important to have an understanding of the normal renal system before understanding any pathology related to this.

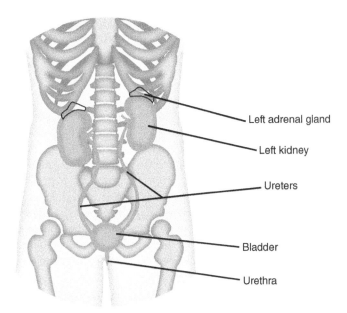

Left adrenal gland

Left kidney

Ureters

Bladder

Urethra

Figure 8.1 The renal system (Cook, 2021)

The main function of the renal system is to excrete waste from the body through the production of urine, which is created in the kidneys. There are usually two kidneys, which are located on each side near the back below the rib cage. Each kidney has a ureter attached which drains the urine produced down to the bladder for storage. Once the bladder starts to become full, nerve endings will signal to the person that it is time to empty the urine. Once the pelvic floor muscles are relaxed, urine will travel down the ureter to exit the body.

There are three internal regions of the kidney (Nagalingham, 2019). The renal cortex contains the capillaries and parts of the nephrons, which is where the filtration and reabsorption occurs. The nephron will be discussed in more detail below. The renal medulla consists of pyramids and is where filtrate is concentrated or diluted. The renal pelvis is where filtrate is funnelled to the ureter. In a healthy human, approximately 625 millilitres of blood will flow through each kidney per minute, which equates to around 25 per cent of cardiac output (Jones and Steggall, 2020).

The ureters are around 30cm long and 5mm in diameter (Nagalingham, 2019). They lead directly from the kidney to the bladder. Urine moves down the ureters through peristalsis, as the ureters are surrounded by muscle.

The bladder is a reservoir for urine that has been produced and is composed of four layers (Jones and Steggall, 2020):

- an outer fibrous adventitia;
- a muscle layer of smooth muscle in inner and outer longitudinal layers with a circular layer, the detrousor, which contracts during micturition;
- a submucosal layer of connective tissue;
- a mucosal layer of transitional epithelium.

Muscles and fibres within the bladder stretch as it fills, transmitting signals to the surrounding sympathetic and parasympathetic nerves.

The urethra leads from the bladder for urine to be excreted. In women this is around 4cm and in men around 20cm (Jones and Steggall, 2020). The top of the urethra has two sphincter muscles. The first, closest to the bladder, is called the internal urethral sphincter, which is smooth muscle in men and smooth muscle with elastic tissue in women, responding to parasympathetic and sympathetic stimulation. This relaxes once the bladder has around 300mls inside, providing the urge to pass urine. The external urethral sphincter is made from skeletal muscle in men and striated muscle in women, which makes it under voluntary control. This is the muscle we relax when ready to pass urine.

The nephron

Urine is produced through the process of filtration. This occurs in nephrons within the kidney. Arterial blood entering the renal artery will split into smaller vessels before passing through the afferent arteriole to the glomerulus, which is within the Bowman's capsule (Jones and Steggall, 2020). Waste products smaller than 7 nanometres will pass through holes called fenestrations. The blood flow will continue through the glomerulus and exit at the efferent arteriole into the renal vein. The waste products will enter the proximal convoluted tubule, through the loop of Henle, into the distal convoluted tubule, then into a collecting tubule before leading down into the ureter to the bladder. See below for each section of the nephron and its role (Nagalingham, 2019; Jones and Steggall, 2020):

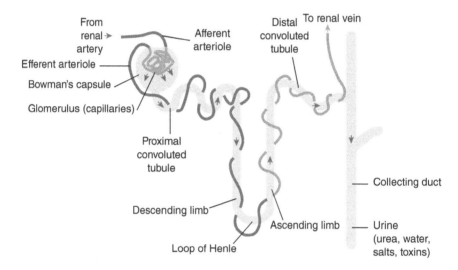

Figure 8.2   The nephron (Cook, 2021)

- glomerulus – a network of capillaries within the Bowman's capsule that filter the blood to remove waste products;
- proximal convoluted tubule (PCT) – reabsorption of glucose, amino acids, metabolites and electrolytes into the circulation. Filtrate continues to the loop of Henle;
- loop of Henle – a large loop connecting the PCT and DCT. Further concentration of the filtrate happens here, reabsorbing fluid or diluting as necessary;
- distal convoluted tubule (DCT) – filtrate continues up the DCT and enters the collecting duct;
- collecting duct – the collecting duct releases the filtrate, now urine, to the ureter.

Pathophysiology of AKI

The pathophysiology can be split into three areas; pre-renal, renal/intra-renal and post-renal (Jones and Steggall, 2020). The causes of each are complex, therefore explained in more depth in each area.

Pre-renal

This indicates that the problem has not originated in the kidney and the AKI is a secondary event. It has been caused by reduced blood flow to the kidney due to another condition. This leads to decreased perfusion of the glomerulus and decreased perfusion of the kidneys. The kidneys receive around 20–25 per cent of cardiac output in a healthy individual. For a period of time, the kidneys will compensate if less perfusion is received; however, decreased perfusion for a prolonged period will lead to damage of the surrounding tissues, causing an intra renal injury (Nagalingham, 2019).

Pre-renal causes of acute kidney injury include hypovolaemia, decreased cardiac output, decreased vascular resistance and decreased cardiovascular blood flow. These are examined in more detail below:

hypovolaemia – most likely causes are dehydration, haemorrhage, GI losses such as diarrhoea and vomiting, or burns;

decreased cardiac output – most likely causes are dysrhythmias, cardiogenic shock, heart failure and myocardial infarction (MI);

decreased peripheral vascular resistance – causes include anaphylaxis and septic shock;

decreased cardiovascular blood flow – most likely caused an embolus.

Renal or intra-renal

These causes are through direct damage to the kidney. Acute tubular necrosis accounts for the vast majority of this category. Acute tubular necrosis is injury to the epithelial cells, which in turn causes renal dysfunction. Less likely causes include renal ischaemia and glomerulonephritis.

Post-renal

These are caused by an obstruction to stop the passage of urine. This could be through a renal calculi, which is the most common, a tumour or an enlarged prostate. Reduction of the obstruction will resolve the AKI.

It is helpful to apply this knowledge to our case study; this is considered for Dilys in the following case study.

Activity 8.2   Evidence-based practice and research

In the case study, Dilys was diagnosed with an AKI. Do you think Dilys experienced a pre-renal, intra-renal or post-renal AKI? Explain why have you chosen this answer.

An outline answer is given at the end of this chapter.

The role of the nursing associate in assessing the patient with AKI

The NA should support the registered nurse (RN) in a variety of ways. The assessment of Dilys is a priority, with the ABCDE approach being most relevant (RCUK, 2021b). This will be completed in

A&E when she is first assessed; however, continued monitoring will ensure that any improvement or deterioration is quickly noted and acted upon whilst she is on the medical ward. The ABCDE approach is shown below in relation to Dilys:

Airway – depending on other conditions present, there may be an issue with consciousness and airway management. An example is severe sepsis. Dilys is able to maintain her own airway with no issue of note;

Breathing – shortness of breath may be evident as the patient may be hyperventilating in an attempt to rid the body of carbon dioxide to correct acidosis. Dilys is tachypnoeic on her initial vital sign monitoring. This would need to be monitored through her admission to ensure any increase or decrease in her respiratory rate is noted in a timely manner. Her saturations were normal on her initial vital signs assessment, but as she has heart failure, her saturations are at risk of reducing, particularly if she develops pulmonary oedema through fluid overload;

Circulation – blood pressure may be low if there is a lack of volume in circulating blood or high if the patient is overloaded with fluid. Manual pulse is important as there is a need to assess the strength of the pulse. A thread weak pulse would indicate a low circulating volume. This is also better practice as you will be able to note any arrhythmias in rate. Reduced urine output will be likely and possibly no output if severe. Dilys was tachycardic initially as well as having AF. Patients with AF should have their pulse rate monitored manually only over one minute due to the irregularity. She was placed on a cardiac monitor, which should be ongoing on the medical ward as she is at risk of arrhythmias secondary to her hyperkalemia. A fluid monitoring chart should be commenced in order for anyone caring for Dilys to be aware of whether there is a positive or negative fluid balance and alter treatment accordingly;

Disability – monitor conscious level. High levels of urea can lead to changes in conscious level. Dilys has been alert throughout but worsening of her condition may present in decreased conscious level;

Exposure – skin rashes are sometimes present in an AKI. Oedema may be present in patients who have fluid overload. As Dilys has heart failure, she is at risk of fluid overload due to medication changes and fluid resuscitation for the AKI. She does not have any rashes on admission to the ward.

Priorities of care for Dilys

The priorities for care for patients with AKI such as Dilys can be identified as preventing it worsening, and maintaining an accurate fluid balance.

Dilys was admitted with several nursing problems, some of which can be reviewed below:

1. shortness of breath – related to fluid overload from the heart failure and also the AKI. She presented tachypnoeic, which is ongoing;
2. oliguria – related to reduced kidney function. Demonstrated through raised creatinine levels compared to previous blood results taken;
3. hyperkalemia – raised potassium noted on initial VBG and also blood tests. Likely secondary to AKI or heart failure. This could have potentially caused the AKI by reducing creatinine clearance.

It is important to consider the nursing goals for Dilys as well as the medical problems in order to provide safe and effective care:

1. restore normal respiration rate – once respiration rate has fallen to within normal parameters, and normal parameters of saturations are maintained;
2. restore normal urine output – ensure that Dilys is producing over 30mls per hour of urine and this is maintained. Maintain a fluid balance chart to document her input and output;
3. restore potassium level to normal parameters – provide treatment for hyperkalemia to restore normal levels within the blood. Review bloods following each treatment to reassess and provide further treatment as prescribed.

STOP AKI is an acronym developed by the Royal College of Physicians (2015a) to help manage patients with an AKI. This can be broken down into:

sepsis;

toxins;

optimise blood pressure;

prevent harm.

For sepsis, the sepsis screening and action tool (Sepsis Trust, 2022) should be initiated; this can be known as the sepsis 6. This is applying high flow oxygen, providing IV fluids, blood tests including haemoglobin, lactate and blood cultures, urine output monitoring and antibiotics. Toxins would be any nephrotoxic medications being administered to the patient, reviewing and holding or stopping these and considering alternatives. See pharmacology below for nephrotoxic medications. Optimising blood pressure would be increasing hypotension to a normal range or reducing hypertension to a normal range. This could be by encouraging fluid intake or omitting certain medications. Preventing harm encourages the review of the cause of the AKI and treating it early. This prevents any further damage occurring and increases the likelihood of clinical improvement back to baseline.

It is important for patients with an AKI to have strict fluid balance monitoring. Any fluid given to the patient or taken orally should be clearly documented, and output should be accurately recorded. This allows for an accurate review of how well the kidneys are able to produce urine as well as monitoring whether the patient has a positive or negative fluid balance. In patients who are dehydrated, the use of a fluid balance is key to note the fluid intake and monitor the fluid status. The patient should be catheterised in order to accurately monitor urine output on an hourly basis. Depending on the electrolyte levels, a fluid restriction may be in place in order to regulate sodium levels. Sodium intake should be monitored and fluid intake based on the previous day's urine output.

When monitoring fluid balance, if the input is less than the output, this is a negative fluid balance. This can indicate that the patient is dehydrated. If input is more than the output, this is a positive fluid balance. This means the patient is overhydrated and is at risk of developing pulmonary oedema. As well as a fluid balance chart, it may be useful to complete a food chart to monitor how much they are eating as well as drinking.

In addition to these priorities, other investigations and aspects of care are also important. It would be useful for a minimum of daily blood tests, in particular urea and electrolytes (U&Es) which will advise the current creatinine levels. Having daily blood tests will monitor whether high creatinine levels are falling, staying the same or increasing. This will provide medical staff with the data to monitor whether the AKI is improving, staying the same or worsening.

Vital signs monitoring is important. This should be completed as per the needs of the patient, as advised by National Early Warning Score (NEWS2) (Royal College of Physicians, 2017) or request of the nurse or medical team caring for the patient. Daily weights may or may not be required in order to monitor fluid retention/overload, particularly in patients who have a cardiac history.

The patient may need an X-ray or an ultrasound of their kidneys, urethra and bladder (KUB) should the AKI be severe or a post-renal cause be suspected. This can provide information such as kidney size and structure and identify renal calculi and the size and position of these. An MRI may be required should a tumour be identified on previous radiological tests in order to provide more characteristics of the tissue and stage the tumour appropriately.

Urinalysis should be performed, should the patient be passing urine. Urine osmolarity may also be requested. The first void sample in the morning is the best for these tests if this is possible to obtain.

Regular electrocardiogram (ECG) monitoring may be indicated if the patient has hyperkalemia. There are often changes to the T wave, making it tall and narrow compared to a normal trace. Regular tracings can monitor for any cardiac arrhythmias that could arise due to the increase in potassium. In severe cases, a patient can have asystole, ventricular fibrillation (VF) or ventricular tachycardia (VT).

Management of the patient with AKI

The NA will work within a multidisciplinary team and with a RN. The RN will review the patient monitoring information provided by the NA, and review the plan of care on a regular basis to ensure that the patient is receiving the correct level of care and support. The care plan should be amended with any improvement or deterioration, highlighting how to continue improvement.

Patients should be assessed regularly using the ABCDE assessment framework and any changes immediately reported to the medical team. Vital signs should be recorded on a regular basis to monitor for any changes in condition, whether these be improvements or deterioration. Any deterioration in fluid balance, urine output, blood pressure or any evidence of sepsis should be immediately communicated to the medical team. The SBAR (situation, background, assessment, recommendations) approach should be used to hand over effectively (Tait and Hansen, 2016).

Severe cases of AKI may require renal replacement therapy, or dialysis. This would be if the patient was critically unwell and kidney function was very poor. A nephrologist would review the patient alongside critical care, who will make the decision on whether this is the correct treatment (NICE, 2019b).

Health promotion

It is important that the nursing associate can identify patients who are at risk of an AKI and provide the relevant health promotion to them. Making patients and their carers aware if they are at risk will allow them to take steps to prevent an AKI from developing. This could be by ensuring patients stay hydrated. In the case of Dilys, she did not want to drink as she had poor mobility due to arthritis and didn't want to keep mobilising to the toilet with urinary urgency. By educating her about her increased risk due to her health conditions and age, she may not have developed the AKI. Informing her during her admission may prevent a recurrence, although having an AKI previously would increase her risk of developing the condition again (NICE, 2019b). Regular GP follow-up to review medication and condition could prevent worsening of heart failure and changes to medication dosage can be changed to prevent nephrotoxicity.

Pharmacology causes of AKI

The long-term use of nephrotoxic medication without adequate monitoring can cause an AKI. There are many nephrotoxic medications. Here are several medication groups:

angiotensin converting enzyme (ACE) inhibitors – ACE inhibitors are used for the treatment of hypertension and heart failure. They are a common medication used for these conditions, such as lisinopril, perindopril and ramipril. Prolonged use can cause AKI and CKD as they are nephrotoxic. Prior to commencing these medications or altering the dosage, renal function should be checked and monitored on a regular basis. Hyperkalemia is common with patients with an impaired renal function who are taking ACE inhibitors. The elderly are at particular risk of this. In patients with an AKI, these should be stopped and an alternative sought (BNF, 2022a);

non-steroidal anti-inflammatory drugs (NSAIDs) – NSAIDs are a large group of medications used for analgesia and anti-inflammatory effects. These include over the counter preparations, such as ibuprofen and prescribed alternatives such as diclofenac, naproxen and mefanamic acid. NSAIDs used over a prolonged period of time can lead to AKI among many other side effects. The link to AKI and NSAIDs is more common when a patient also has an increased alcohol consumption. These medications are usually only for short-term use, but as ibuprofen can be bought over the counter, many patients may not realise this, should they not read the information leaflet. Highlight to the registered nurse and the medical team caring for the patient if you notice they have prolonged use of NSAIDs and/or have a high alcohol consumption (BNF, 2022b);

Should a patient be taking NSAIDs and ACE inhibitors at the same time, they are at increased risk of hyperkalemia.

metformin – metformin is mainly prescribed for the control of blood glucose in diabetic patients, but it can also be used for treatment of polycystic ovaries. Metformin should not be prescribed for patients with an estimated glomerular filtration rate (eGFR) of 30 or less due to the nephrotoxicity of the medication. Use in patients with an impaired kidney function can lead to AKI (BNF, 2022c);

loop diuretics – loop diuretics include medications such as furosemide, bumetanide and co-amilofruse. Loop diuretics inhibit the reabsorption from the loop of Henle, making them potent diuretics. They are contra indicated in patients who have renal failure secondary to nephrotoxic medication. Taking these medications whilst having an AKI can be detrimental and should be stopped until the AKI has been resolved (BNF, 2022a).

Pharmacology for treatment of AKI

In treating an AKI, there is a requirement to normalise any hyperkalemia and ensure that dehydration is treated. Dehydration would be treated with intravenous fluids. Dilys has heart failure with oedema, so intravenous fluids should be prescribed over a greater length of time to prevent further oedema occurring. Hyperkalemia would be treated with calcium gluconate and an insulin – glucose infusion with regular blood tests after each set of treatment until the range returned to normal. It is useful to review this pharmacology in relation to Dilys; this is considered in the following activity.

Activity 8.3   Critical thinking

In the case study, Dilys was prescribed ramipril, furosemide and naproxen prior to her admission. What would you do if you were caring for Dilys and saw these medications prescribed on her medication chart?

An outline answer is provided at the end of the chapter.

Chapter summary

This chapter began with a case study, which identified a patient, Dilys, admitted to hospital with an AKI. Throughout the chapter, there has been discussion around the symptoms, pathophysiology, assessment and management of the condition. There was consideration around the condition itself and how it links to other conditions and can be a secondary diagnosis. Activities throughout will have helped you to link the literature to the case study and help recognise how an AKI can affect a patient in your care.

Activities: brief outline answers

Activity 8.1 Critical thinking

Dilys has several pre-existing conditions that would put her at increased risk of developing an AKI. She is over the age of 65, has a heart failure diagnosis, has attended with oliguria and is taking several nephrotoxic medications. As she is taking furosemide, a loop diuretic, she is not drinking as much as she needs to pass urine often, which has led to dehydration.

Activity 8.2 Evidence-based practice and research

The main cause is pre-renal; reduced blood flow to the kidneys. This is usually secondary to another health condition. In the case of Dilys, she had heart failure, where many of these symptoms are similar in presentation. She was dehydrated due to her lack of fluid intake, and the combination of this and being prescribed numerous nephrotoxic medications meant it was inevitable she was going to develop an AKI. Patients rarely attend hospital/GP for AKI only. Reduced blood flow can be due to anaemia, severe dehydration, heart failure, sepsis, vascular disease and medications that are nephrotoxic. Many of these factors are evidenced within the case study of Dilys as outlined above.

Activity 8.3 Critical thinking

Dilys has many risk factors, making her high risk of developing an AKI. When a patient is already high risk and has many nephrotoxic medications charted, this should be brought to the attention of the medical team caring for her so they can consider alternatives.

Do not withhold medication without discussing this with the medical team as this could potentially cause further harm and deteriorate her condition further.

Further reading

Andrade, M. and Knight, J. (2017) Anatomy and Physiology of aging 4: the renal system. Available at: https://cdn.ps.emap.com/wp-content/uploads/sites/3/2017/05/046-049_PrSoLRenal4_030517-KJCT.pdf

Useful article on changes to the renal system as patients are aging.

KDIGO (2012) Acute Kidney Injury. Available at: https://kdigo.org/guidelines/acute-kidney-injury/

KDIGO Guidelines for AKI.

Useful website

https://britishrenal.org/ – British Renal Society

This website considers all aspects of kidney damage, but has specific sections and guidelines on patients with an AKI.

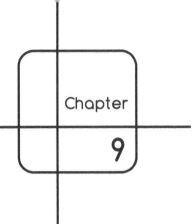

Chapter 9

The acutely ill trauma patient: road traffic accident (RTA)

Laura Whitehead

(Continued)

3.16   demonstrate the ability to recognise the effects of medicines, allergies, drug sensitivity, side-effects, contraindications and adverse reactions

Chapter aims

By the end of this chapter, you will be able to:

- define what is meant by the term trauma and discuss the different types of trauma-associated injuries;
- understand how to assess a trauma patient, including the primary and secondary survey;
- explain the complications associated with trauma, including the various types and management of shock;
- discuss the management of a trauma patient, including pharmacological interventions and the monitoring required.

Introduction

Trauma is one of the biggest killers in the United Kingdom (NICE, 2016b). Major trauma is defined as serious multiple injuries that require lifesaving interventions (NICE, 2016b). People under the age of 20 and over 65 are statistically more likely to suffer from major trauma, and trauma is the biggest killer of people below the age of 45 (NICE, 2016b). Every year in England and Wales 16,000 people die after sustaining a trauma-related injury, with millions more acquiring non-fatal injuries (Trauma & Audit Research Network, 2022). In the last 25 years, however, there has been an improvement in outcomes for patients. This is due to advancements in prehospital and A&E care and management (NICE, 2016b).

The Trauma Audit Research Network (TARN) collects data on trauma patients and their outcomes. This enables us to understand the benefits and risks associated with treatment and injuries (TARN, 2022). By auditing hospitals in England and Wales, variations in treatment and outcomes can be established which provides a unique opportunity to improve care (TARN, 2022). TARN is an example of how audit and data collection impacts on the quality of patient care.

In 2011 the Regional Trauma Networks were established in England and Wales (NHS Clinical Advisory Group on Trauma, 2010). The network was set up to ensure that people with major trauma were treated in hospitals which have appropriately trained staff that can provide timely care (NICE, 2016b). Trauma centres specialise in caring for people with trauma injuries. At the centre of the trauma network is the major trauma centre. This is a hospital that has multiple specialities on one site, to ensure trauma care is efficient and consultant-level care is provided (NICE, 2016b).

This chapter will outline the types of injuries a trauma patient might suffer from. It will focus on an acutely ill trauma patient, using a case study and self-directed activities. A rolling case study will be used throughout, so you will be provided with new information about the patient and their journey from the roadside, to A&E and eventually theatre. There will be a focus on the primary and secondary survey of this patient. The patient, Andrzej, was admitted following a road traffic accident with a compound fracture and hypovolaemic shock. Throughout the self-directed activities you will identify the key nursing problems and the priorities of care. You will follow this patient through to Chapter 10, where Andrzej will develop post-operative complications following repair of the compound fracture.

Defining trauma

There are different types of trauma, with different mechanisms of injury. People can have a variety of injuries as a result of trauma that require specialist input and care. Trauma is defined as blunt, penetrating force or perforating injury which occurs to the body and results in injury (Tait et al., 2016):

- *blunt injury* can be caused by a fall or a seat belt injury which leaves the skin intact but can cause internal injuries (Tait et al., 2016);
- *penetrating trauma* is an injury where the body surface is damaged, for example due to a stab injury, where the skin is broken and there is damage to the tissues beneath (Tait et al., 2016). This could be caused by a knife or a glass bottle.
- *a perforating injury* which occurs when an object passes through the body and leaves an entrance and exit wound (Bersten and Soni, 2013). An example of a perforating injury would be a gun shot, which can pass through the body and damage whatever tissue it passes through.

Case study: Andrzej, the acutely ill trauma patient

Andrzej is a 40-year-old man, admitted to A&E following a road traffic accident (RTA). Andrzej was driving his car at approximately 60 miles per hour (mph) when a car pulled out from a side road, giving Andrzej little opportunity to stop. It took a while for the emergency services to cut Andrzej from the car and stabilise his right femur open fracture. On arrival at A&E, Andrzej has cervical spine (c-spine) immobilisation, and his observations are:

- heart rate (HR): 135 beats per minute (bpm);
- blood pressure (BP): 85/65 millimetres of mercury (mmHg);
- respiratory rate (RR): >25 breaths per minute (bpm);
- saturations (SpO2): 93%;
- temperature (TEMP): 35.5 °C;
- GCS 14/15 – Andrzej is slightly disoriented/confused.

The paramedic handed over that Andrzej had lost about 1 litre of blood from the open compound fracture. On transit to A&E Andrzej received 1 litre of 0.9 per cent normal saline, 1 litre of oxygen via nasal cannula, paracetamol intravenous (IV) and 2mgs of IV morphine for pain, and he has two large bore cannulas inserted. Andrzej's next of kin is his wife; she has been notified by the police and is on her way to the hospital.

(Continued)

(Continued)

This case study of Andrzej is used throughout this chapter, and also in Chapters 10 and 11, showing how his care is managed in different areas in relation to his acute needs.

Trauma care pathway

It is important that trauma patients are assessed using a systematic approach. They can have a range of injuries from single organ damage to multiple complex injuries that require timely intervention from a variety of healthcare professionals in different disciplines (Adam et al., 2017).

Care of the person with traumatic injuries begins in the prehospital setting. Trauma patients are assessed using a primary and secondary survey approach. Initial management is focused on life-threatening issues and maintenance of the airway, breathing and circulation (Adam et al., 2017).

As part of the care provided it is important that it is identified which hospital the patient is taken to to receive treatment. This decision will be based on the location and type of injuries the person has. Due to Andrzej sustaining complex injuries he was brought into a major trauma centre A&E by ambulance. A major trauma centre specialises in looking after people with injuries like Andrzej's so he will have specialists providing expert input on his care. On arrival at A&E it is vital that Andrzej receives timely care; in order for this to occur Andrzej must first be assessed. See the diagram in Figure 9.1 which explains the stages that occur in the trauma pathway.

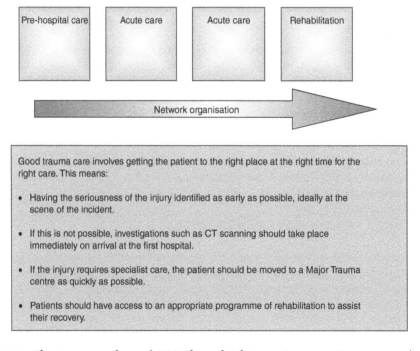

Figure 9.1 The trauma pathway (NHS Clinical Advisory Group on Trauma, 2010)

Activity 9.1   Critical thinking

- What assessment approach should be used when assessing Andrzej?
- Why is this the chosen assessment approach?

An outline answer is provided at the end of this chapter.

Assessing the trauma patient

There are four stages of assessment which occur with a trauma patient:

- primary survey;
- resuscitation phase;
- secondary phase;
- definitive care plan.

Primary survey

The aim of a primary survey is to identify and treat any life-threatening issues or conditions that a trauma patient may have. This is done by using an ABCDE approach (RCUK, 2021b). This assessment considers airway, breathing, circulation, disability and dysfunction and exposure, and will have been carried out by the paramedics at the scene of the incident and will be carried out again once the patient has arrived in A&E. It is vital as part of this primary survey that the patient is continuously reassessed – this is to ensure that any deterioration is noticed early so interventions can be implemented as a matter of urgency (Adam et al., 2017). For a primary survey of the trauma patient an ABCDE assessment (RCUK, 2021b) is carried out; however, there are some additional components to the assessment that are required for a trauma patient that you may not have seen or carried out before.

Airway maintenance and cervical spine control: From using a look, listen and feel approach (RCUK, 2021c) we know that Andrzej is maintaining his own airway and is talking, there are no signs of airway obstruction and there are no additional sounds. You should look inside Andrzej's mouth: are there any blood clots, vomit, teeth or debris present? If so these need to be removed. When someone is a trauma patient, management of their cervical spine is done at the same time as that of their airway. If a neck injury is a possibility then precautions must be taken with the patient's cervical spine. From the scenario we know that Andrzej has his c-spine immobilised. This is because he was involved in a high-speed car accident, which makes him at risk of having injured his spine. It is important that Andrzej's neck is not hyperextended as this could cause further injury. Andrzej will need to have his cervical spine assessed; this will be done by a senior medical or nursing colleague. They will assess Andrzej to see whether he has any neck pain on palpation, and further imaging (such as X-ray or CT scan) may be needed to rule out any injury. Until the c-spine can be cleared, precautions need to stay in place – we call this c-spine immobilisation. This is why Andrzej is still wearing a neck brace, has been told to remain very still and has blocks either side of his head to keep his neck in line and immobilised.

Breathing and ventilation: Andrzej's chest would need to be exposed to assess respiratory movement. Andrzej's oxygen saturations are 93 per cent, therefore oxygen has been administered via a nasal cannula by the paramedics. However, as he is a trauma patient and there is a risk of deterioration, high flow oxygen would be administered via a 15L non-rebreathe mask

Adam et al., 2017). His respiratory rate is greater than 25 – he is tachypnoeic. His chest is clear, there are no added sounds. He would need to be assessed to see whether there is equal rise and fall of the chest. There are no signs of central or peripheral cyanosis. Due to Andrzej being involved in a car accident and the fact that he was wearing a seat belt, he requires a chest X-ray to see if he has a blunt chest injury. The chest X-ray was NAD (nothing abnormal detected).

Circulation and haemorrhage control: It is vital that Andrzej's haemodynamic status is determined. Vital signs such as blood pressure, heart rate, skin colour and capillary refill must be done as a matter of urgency. Andrzej is hypotensive with a blood pressure of 85/65mmHg and has had a litre of fluid in the ambulance. He has an estimated blood loss (EBL) of 1 litre and is still losing blood from the open wound on his leg. A crossmatch blood sample and a group and save would need to be taken from Andrzej. These blood tests determine what blood group Andrzej has so if he needs a transfusion the correct blood group can be administered. From the scenario, the most obvious source of blood loss is the open fracture; however, Andrzej will need a pelvis X-ray and ultrasound scans called eFAST (extended focused assessment with sonography for trauma) (NICE, 2016b). An eFAST scan is an ultrasound scan which is used to determine whether there are sources of active bleeding in trauma patients; the scan should be used alongside further assessment of the patient (NICE, 2016b) and is normally carried out by a senior medical or nursing colleague. He is tachycardic with a heart rate of 135bpm and hypothermic with a temperature of 35.5°C. He has an open fracture; his peripheries are cool to touch but a pulse is present in all of his limbs.

From these observations we know that Andrzej is acutely unwell and is showing signs of being in shock. As per the National Institute for Clinical Excellence guidelines on *Major Trauma: Asessment and Initial Management* (2016b), as Andrzej is showing signs of shock and he is still actively bleeding he requires an urgent blood transfusion. Emergency blood is available in A&E; trauma patients who receive unmatched blood (as we do not know what blood group Andrzej has) will receive Type O Rh-negative (Rh-) blood until their blood group is known and they can have matched blood (Miraflor et al., 2012).

To receive this blood Andrzej will also need to have peripheral intravenous access (cannula) inserted for when intravenous medications need to be administered. He will also need a full set of blood tests taken, full blood count, urea and electrolytes, coagulation screen, troponin, cross match and group and save. A venous blood gas can also be taken at this time and run through the blood gas machine; this will give you some blood results very quickly and can help when planning the next interventions that Andrzej requires.

Disability – dysfunction of the nervous system and neurological status: A rapid assessment of Andrzej's neurological function must be carried out as soon as possible. Andrzej has a reduced level of consciousness with a Glasgow Coma Score (Teasdale, 2014) of 14/15 due to confusion and disorientation. It is important to see whether Andrzej is orientated to person, time and place. Ensure you are reorienting Andrzej as to where is he and what is happening. As Andrzej has been involved in a car crash there is a risk that he may have a head injury; therefore his level of consciousness will need to be assessed regularly and documented (Teasdale, 2014). Andrzej's pupils will need to be assessed, by shining a light into each of them and seeing whether his pupils are reactive. If the reaction is normal, sluggish or there is no reaction, this needs to be documented. Any changes in pupillary reaction need to be communicated to a senior member of the multidisciplinary team as a matter of urgency. Should the pupils become sluggish or non-reactive this is a sign that there is raised pressure within the brain (intra cranial pressure) and is an emergency. Andrzej's pain score needs to be assessed – make sure that you are using an assessment method appropriate for the patient, their level of consciousness and ability to communicate (NICE, 2016b).

Exposure: Andrzej's clothes were removed and a full body assessment of his injuries was carried out. Privacy and dignity were maintained throughout this assessment (NMC, 2018d). As Andrzej has a low temperature it is important that he is not left undressed too long as this will reduce his temperature further. Ensure that his injuries are documented in his notes – this will help with the secondary survey, which will be discussed later on in the chapter.

Activity 9.2   Critical thinking

From the primary survey above what do you think are the most urgent issues?
An outline answer is provided at the end of this chapter.

Resuscitation phase

Throughout the primary survey, interventions were implemented that aim to stabilise Andrzej's clinical condition (Adam et al., 2017). In the resuscitation phase the management of shock needs to be continued alongside reassessing Andrzej's oxygenation and haemorrhage control. During this phase Andrzej will also require a urinary catheter to be inserted; this is to accurately monitor his urine output (Adam et al., 2017). Currently Andrzej has lost 1000mls of blood; however, should this increase to 1500–2000mls then the hospital major bleeding protocol needs to be activated. When this protocol is activated, O-negative blood, fresh frozen plasma and platelets become available as a matter of urgency (Adam et al., 2017). As per the NICE guidelines (2016b), when a trauma patient is actively bleeding and showing signs of shock for every unit of red blood cells administered, a unit of clotting factor such as fresh frozen plasma and platelets should be administered too. This is because the patient is losing not only red blood cells but also clotting factors as well. During the resuscitation phase, any of the life-threatening conditions that were identified and highlighted during the primary survey need to be constantly reassessed, even when management and interventions are being implemented (Adam et al., 2017). Andrzej will need to have his vital signs monitored every 15 minutes (Royal College of Physicians, 2017), along with a strict fluid balance being recorded with hourly urine output monitoring.

Shock

Shock is a life-threatening condition and the patient needs urgent intervention. Shock is caused by circulatory failure, where tissues do not have enough oxygen (Alexiou and Rau, 2022). There are different types of shock which have different causes. If left untreated the lack of oxygen to the tissues can cause multi-organ failure and lead to death (Alexiou and Rau, 2022).

When a person is in shock this results in a lack of oxygen delivery to the tissues; this can be caused by a low cardiac output, lack of haemoglobin (remember that each haemoglobin cell carried four oxygen molecules, so if there is low haemoglobin due to haemorrhage then the patient may also have hypoxia and hypoxemia) or the ability of the cell to use the oxygen, which is impacted by the cell's ability to generate energy in the form of ATP (adenosine triphosphate) (Adam et al., 2017). Regardless of the cause or the type of shock the person is experiencing, their body will try and compensate in order to maintain homeostasis; if the cause of the shock is not addressed this will lead to multi-organ failure (Tait et al., 2016).

There are different types of shock in different categories, depending on the underlying cause:

- *Cardiogenic shock* due to impaired cardiac function. It is caused by decreased right or left ventricle pump function. This is usually due to injury to the myocardium (this is caused by ischemia which occurs in a myocardial infarction or myocarditis) (Tait et al., 2016). It can also be as a result of structural defects in the heart, cardiac arrythmias and myocardial contusion (bruising of the heart) (Tait et al., 2016). The patient might be bradycardiac or tachycardic, hypotensive or present with low cardiac output. The cause of the cardiogenic shock needs to be identified – this might be through clinical assessment, blood tests (troponin), ECGs, ultrasound of the heart and the patient's past medical history. Treatment depends on the cause; if the patient is suspected of having myocardial infarction then they will treated on the Acute Coronary Syndrome pathway.

- *Inflammatory shock* occurs due to a generalised inflammatory response that leads to organ failure. Sepsis is the main cause of inflammatory shock and is a life-threatening condition that occurs when the body has an abnormal response to an infection (UK Sepsis Trust, 2020). Sepsis can be caused by any bacteria, fungi or viruses (UK Sepsis Trust, 2020). The most common cause of sepsis is pneumonia; however, the other leading causes are gastrointestinal pathology, urinary tract, biliary tract and skin infections (UK Sepsis Trust, 2020). The inflammation caused by sepsis leads to hypotension, vasodilation and myocardial depression (Adam et al., 2017). The patient will need to be treated as per the sepsis guidelines (NICE, 2020b). The patient with suspected sepsis will need to have an immediate review by a senior colleague (NICE, 2020b). Blood tests will need to be done, including blood cultures, venous blood gas, full blood count, C-reactive protein, urea and electrolytes, creatinine and a clotting screen (NICE, 2020b). Broad spectrum antibiotics should be given within an hour of identifying that the patient is high risk; a bolus of IV fluid should also be administered (NICE, 2017b). High risk patients should be monitored every half hour along with their vital signs – the patient's mental state and level of consciousness should be assessed and any changes need to be discussed with a consultant as a matter of urgency (NICE, 2017c).

- *Hypovolemic shock* occurs due to a decreased circulatory volume. This can occur as a result of excess fluid loss due to haemorrhage, vomiting, burns or inadequate fluid intake (Adam et al., 2017). The person might have decreased blood or plasma or extra cellular fluid volume (Tait et al., 2016). This leads to organ hypo-perfusion, which the body will initially try to compensate for by increasing the patient's heart rate; if the hypovolaemia is not corrected or if the person continues to lose fluid they will have a reduced cardiac output (Tait et al., 2016). It is important that the cause of the hypovolaemia is identified and corrected – the patient may require blood transfusion and surgery.

- *Anaphylactic shock* occurs after a potentially life-threatening reaction to an antigen. The reaction normally happens very shortly after exposure to the antigen; the antigens which cause the reaction can vary according to the person. Anaphylaxis is characterised by a sudden onset and quick progression of symptoms; these include airway and/or breathing and/or circulation problems (RCUK, 2021f). Some patients may have skin changes, they might become flushed, develop urticaria (hives/itchy rash); however, these symptoms might not be obvious and may worsen over time (RCUK, 2021f). A diagnosis of anaphylaxis is supported if the person has been exposed to an antigen that they know they are allergic to; however, in 30 per cent of cases there is no obvious trigger (RCUK, 2021f). If untreated the person will have rapid onset cardiovascular collapse, which can lead to death (Adam et al., 2017). The patient might have already self-administered adrenaline via an epi-pen; intravenous access should be gained as the patient may require further adrenaline depending on their response to the intramuscular adrenaline (RCUK, 2021f).

- *Neurogenic shock* may occur in patients with cervical or high thoracic spinal cord injury who develop symptoms of shock due to changes in their sympathetic nervous system. The person develops hypotension and bradycardia and is unable to control their body temperature (Sagar and Cho, 2022). This is due to the sudden loss of sympathetic tone which leans to instability of the autonomic nervous system (Sagar and Cho, 2022). It needs to be managed aggressively with intravenous fluids and vasopressors to maintain an adequate blood pressure to ensure that further secondary injury to the spinal cord doesn't happen (Sagar and Cho, 2022).

- *Obstructive shock* is when an obstruction occurs that blocks or disrupts blood flow from a vessel or within the heart. This can be caused by a pulmonary embolus, tension pneumothorax or pericardial tamponade (Adam et al., 2017). Pericardial tamponade occurs when a build-up of blood or fluid in the pericardial space prevents the ventricles from expanding fully, which decreases ventricular filling (Adam et al., 2017). The septum in the heart ends up bending towards the left ventricle, which decreases the stroke volume and causes obstructive shock; if left untreated it will lead to a cardiac arrest (Adam et al., 2017). Pericardial tamponade can be caused by pericarditis, aortic aneurysm, trauma to the heart, myocardial infarction or heart surgery (Adam et al., 2017). The person might present with hypotension, muffled heart sounds or ST changes on an ECG (Adam et al., 2017). The patient will require a variety of tests including ECGs, echo, angiogram or a CT scan to determine the cause of the obstructive shock. Treatment depends on the cause – if the patient is suspected of having myocardial infarction then they will be treated on the Acute Coronary Syndrome pathway or they may require a percutaneous coronary intervention (NICE, 2020a).

Activity 9.3 Evidence-based practice

What type of shock do you think Andrzej has? What objective data do you have from the scenario and subsequent assessments to support this? How do you think Andrzej should be treated?
An outline answer is provided at the end of this chapter.

Secondary phase

Once the life-threatening conditions have been identified and treated and the treatment for shock has begun, the secondary survey can take place (Adam et al., 2017). The secondary survey includes a detailed and thorough head to toes assessment where every part of the body is examined in detail. Further testing such as X-rays, ultrasound or CT scans occur as part of this stage. The dressing put on by the paramedics is removed so the wound can be assessed carefully. In this survey multiple X-rays are taken of Andrzej's right femur. This exam and imaging take place to ensure that the patient has been assessed to determine whether there are any further injuries that require intervention. Andrzej will also be questioned on his symptoms and his past medical history. The interventions required for Andrzej's specific injuries will be discussed later in the chapter.

Fractures

A fracture is a complete or partial break in a bone. If the skin on top of the bone is intact this is called a closed fracture; if the skin is broken this is called an open or compound fracture (Smith et al., 2016). The term fracture is used to describe a wide range of breaks, all the way from a hairline fracture to a fragmented open fracture (McRae, 2006). Patients with closed fractures may have wounds or breaks in their skin; however, these are not related to the fracture and are superficial (McRae, 2006). In open fractures the broken skin or wound is related to the fracture or break in the bone and patients are at significant risk of infection and haemorrhage (McRae, 2006).

The initial surgical management of the open fracture in theatres will be discussed in detail in the next chapter; however, the section below outlines the interventions that would occur in A&E.

Initial management of open fractures

- A wound swab should be taken to find out whether there are any bacteria in the wound.
- Antibiotics should be considered due to the infection risk (NICE, 2017a).

- The wound should be covered with a saline soaked dressing prior to the patient going to theatre. This is to reduce the risk of hospital-acquired infection (McRae, 2006).
- A temporary plaster back slab should be applied to the limb to provide support until the patient goes to theatre (McRae, 2006).

The prescriber may need to liaise with microbiology as to the most suitable antibiotic for Andrzej; the swab should be taken prior to the administration of antibiotics if possible. Many members of the multidisciplinary team working in A&E are trained in applying casts. This might include nurses, nursing associates, healthcare assistants and plaster technicians. Andrzej will need analgesia prior to the cast being applied, so it is vital that that a comprehensive pain assessment has been carried out and that his pain is reassessed throughout the procedure (NICE, 2017a). The open wound also needs to be dressed with a sterile dressing, including saline soaked gauze (NICE, 2017a) – ensure that an aseptic non-touch technique is used.

Case study: Andrzej (continued)

Andrzej will be having surgery to repair the bone; depending on the type of open fracture, debridement of the wound and skin might be required. Surgery, including fixation to repair and cover the fractured bone, should occur within 12 hours if it is a high-energy open fracture and 24 hours if it is any other type of open fracture (NICE, 2017a). As Andrzej's was a high-energy open fracture because he was involved in a car accident at speed, the repair would need to occur within 12 hours. If there is a wound over the fracture and this cannot be repaired, negative pressure wound therapy should be considered (NICE, 2017a). The surgery will happen as a matter of urgency due to the infection risk his fracture poses. Andrzej was transferred from A&E to theatres. You will follow Andrzej on this next stage of his journey in the next chapter.

Chapter summary

This chapter has discussed in depth the care of a trauma patient being brought in by ambulance to A&E. You are talked through the primary survey and how it contains additional components when the patient is a trauma patient, from the ABCDE assessment (RCUK, 2021b) that you are familiar with. The assessment and care provided are discussed in detail in the resuscitation phase, with a particular focus on the fact that Andrzej is acutely unwell with shock. Within the secondary survey the assessment and interventions were outlined, which again are altered in a trauma patient. You learned about the different types of shock and what causes them. Andrzej was given a definitive care plan of needing surgery to repair his fracture; he was also acutely unwell and required frequent monitoring and assessment. You have identified what the priorities of care are and how these would be prioritised. The model answers at the end of the chapter should be used to assist you in reflecting on the activities you have completed as you worked through this chapter.

Activities: brief outline answers

Activity 9.1 Critical thinking

An ABCDE assessment (RCUK, 2021b) should be carried out as he is acutely unwell and at risk of deterioration.

Activity 9.2 Critical thinking

Blood loss and hypotension
Open fracture
Hypothermia
Change in level of consciousness
Andrzej is acutely unwell and has developed shock

Activity 9.3 Evidence-based practice

Hypovolaemic shock because he has an estimated blood loss of 1L, he has reduced cardiac output, is tachycardic and hypotensive. There is a clear cause of his hypovolaemia: the open leg fracture.

Andrzej needs to be administered IV fluids or a unit of red blood cells. He needs to go to theatre urgently to repair his fracture. He needs to be continuously assessed, vital signs being recorded every 15 minutes. His level of consciousness needs to be monitored as he has an altered level of consciousness which could be due to the blood loss, the accident or as a result of an infection.

Further reading

Alexiou, A. and Rau, C. (2022) Shock: symptoms, diagnosis and treatment. *British Medical Journal online.* Available at: https://bestpractice.bmj.com/topics/en-gb/3000121 (accessed 6 July 2022)

This article is a comprehensive information source on shock, assessment, diagnosis and management.

Headway (2022) *Brain Injury Association Resources.* Available at: www.headway.org.uk/ (accessed 6 July 2022)

Headway is a charity which supports people and their friends and families who have experienced a brain injury; their website is full of information, resources and advice.

The Trauma Audit Research Network (2022) *TARN Trauma courses.* Available online at: www.tarn.ac.uk/Content.aspx?ca=6 (accessed on 6 July 2022)

The Trauma Audit Research Network is a fantastic resource for learning about trauma and the patient pathway; there are also free e-learning resources available and interactive resources.

United Kingdom Trauma Council (2022) *Resources.* Available at: uktraumacouncil.org (accessed on 6 July 2022)

The UK Trauma Council is another source of useful resources.

Resuscitation Council UK (2021b) ABCDE approach. Available at: www.resus.org.uk/library/abcde-approach (accessed 28 November 2021)

The RCUK has detailed information around patient assessment and interventions.

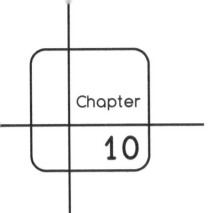

Chapter 10

The acutely ill post-operative patient: post-operative complication

Sinead Mehigan

Chapter aims

By the end of this chapter you will be able to:

- understand what you need to prepare to receive a patient from surgery in the Post Anaesthetic Care Unit (PACU);
- describe the process of safe handover of the patient by the anaesthetist to the PACU team;
- identify the skills required to assess, plan, deliver and evaluate safe care to the patient in the PACU setting;
- discuss some common post-operative complications seen in the PACU.

Introduction

This chapter links with both Chapter 9 and Chapter 11, as it focusses on the ongoing care that one patient, Andrzej, receives at various stages in the treatment of his compound fracture, following an RTA. The focus of care in this chapter is on the immediate post-operative stage. This is immediately after surgery, and takes place in a special unit, sometimes called recovery, but more accurately called the Post Anaesthetic Care Unit (PACU). All patients who have undergone surgery under general, spinal or epidural anaesthesia need to be recovered in a PACU by a nurse or qualified practitioner who has had specific development to be able to do so, until such time as the patient is fit enough to be transferred to a ward area. The standards of care provided in these units have been set out by the Association of Anaesthetists of Great Britain and Ireland (Association of Anaesthetists of Great Britain and Ireland, 2013). The emphasis of care in this area is on maintaining patient safety, through close assessment and monitoring.

This chapter will follow Andrzej, the patient from Chapter 9, who presented following a road traffic accident (RTA). He then had surgery for a repair of a compound fracture. Post-operative complications will be addressed with links to pathophysiology. Assessment of the post-operative patient will be discussed and priorities of care identified. Links to evidence-based practice will be made to justify the management of post-operative complications. The chapter is written practically, and will hopefully give the reader some principles of post-operative care that can be applied to the care of a wide range of post-operative patients. This chapter will lead on to Chapter 11, which focuses on the patient who, following his time in recovery, develops sepsis.

Case study: Andrzej, the acutely ill post-operative patient (continued from Chapter 9)

Following direct transfer from A&E, Andrzej undergoes emergency surgery to debride his wound and to stabilise the compound fracture of his right femur. The surgical team stabilise his fracture by carrying out an Open Reduction and Internal Fixation (ORIF) of his right femur using pin and plate. The team estimate that, between A&E and surgery, he has lost over 1.5 litres of blood.

Once Andrzej's surgery is complete, the anaesthetic team reverse the effects of their anaesthetic agents, so that he begins to wake up in theatre.

Preparing to receive your patient

Prior to receiving any patient to the PACU, it is important that the unit has been prepared – ideally at the beginning of each shift. This includes:

- checking of the resuscitation trolley – and recording that it has been done;
- checking drug and fluid supplies – restocking if necessary;
- restocking all disposables – including those stored by each bed space;
- checking oxygen supplies – including a range of masks and adjuncts and suction equipment are checked and stock replenished by each bed space;
- ensuring each bed space has clean sharps disposal bins and rubbish bags;
- ensuring spare linen, including gowns and blankets for patient warming, are available;
- checking alarm bells first thing in the morning.

Before Andrzej is transferred to the PACU, the nurse or nursing associate who will care for him will need to check the following in the bed space where he will be recovered, and ensure:

- new high capacity sucker is switched on and working;
- oxygen mask is available for immediate use – meaning it is connected;
- additional support for Andrzej's breathing is available if needed – this might be a Hudson mask, or bag-valve-mask device – or an Ambu bag with mask fitted;
- pulse oximeter working and switched on;
- blood pressure monitor is available – along with 3-lead ECG if needed;
- IV drip stand is available.

It is useful to review this process with that in the previous chapter, in the following activity.

Activity 10.1 Reflection

Review the previous chapter where Andrzej was cared for in the A&E department, and reflect on how each area is set up to prepare to receive patients.

What are some of the similarities, and some of the differences?

An outline answer is provided at the end of this chapter.

Initial handover

When a patient is brought into the recovery unit, they must be accompanied by the anaesthetist, and a member of the surgical team (Association of Anaesthetists of Great Britain and Ireland (AAGBI), 2013). The nurse or nursing associate with responsibility for recovering any patient in the PACU should immediately ensure that the patient is appropriately positioned (generally on their side, with the surgical side uppermost) and that they put on an appropriate oxygen mask. A sucker should be turned on and positioned under the patient's pillow. They should check their level of consciousness, and that the patient is stable, and breathing quietly. While they are doing this, another person can put on all monitoring devices, such as pulse oximeter and non-invasive blood pressure cuff, and record their pulse and blood pressure.

Once this is done, and the receiving PACU nurse is confident that the patient is stable, they must then be given a full handover, from both the anaesthetist and the surgical team member accompanying them. This includes the patient's identity, the actual surgery carried out, whether or not there were any complications, whether they had any pre-existing illnesses that might affect their recovery, anaesthetic drugs and IV fluids administered – and, based on blood loss, what future IV fluid requirements are. The anaesthetist should identify what analgesics were given, and what they expect will be needed in the post-operative period. Have there been any issues with nausea and vomiting? Have they ordered antiemetics? They also need to identify how much oxygen the patient needs, and how this should be given, and whether or not they require additional monitoring of the patient while in the unit, or orders for further investigations.

The PACU team should also be given details of vital signs, including pulse, blood pressure and respiration during the procedure. In the case of Andrzej, he will have been given antibiotics in theatre – so the PACU nurse will need to know when the next dose is due. If urine output was measured during the procedure, what was it, and what is the expected output for the next few hours? Are there any drains inserted, and have the surgical and anaesthetic team any specific post-operative instructions?

Case study: Andrzej's initial observations at handover (continued)

- heart rate (HR): 85 beats per minute (bpm);
- blood pressure (BP): 110/65 millimetres of mercury (mmHg);
- respiratory rate (RR): 14 breaths per minute (bpm);
- saturations (SpO2): 96%;
- temperature (TEMP): 36 °C.

The anaesthetist needs to check with the PACU nurse or nursing associate, that they are happy with the handover and the patient's condition, before they leave the unit. Before the anaesthetist leaves, they need to check that the patient's breathing, blood pressure and oxygen saturation are stable. The anaesthetist should also tell the team how they can be contacted, in case the patient deteriorates – they need to remain close to the PACU while their patients are there (AAGBI, 2013).

Principles of nursing assessment in the Post Anaesthetic Care Unit (PACU)

As the anaesthetic team give their handover, the nurse or nursing associate in PACU will make their own systematic assessment of the patient's condition – using a modified form of the ABCDE approach (Hatfield, 2014) that was covered in Chapter 2. This involves assessment, in this order, of:

- A – Airway: Is the patient able to maintain their own airway? Is their airway clear? This can be checked by putting a hand over the patient's mouth for a brief moment to feel whether the air is moving freely, and putting another hand gently on their chest to feel whether it is moving up and down. The most common problem post-operatively is airway obstruction, due to the patient's tongue falling to the back of their throat. You will know this has happened if you hear the patient snoring. If this happens, the patient should be put onto their side (if they are not already). If this is not possible, staff will need to perform a 'chin lift'. It could also be that a patient has mucous at the back of their throat, leading to a gurgling sound. This can be resolved by gently suctioning secretions from the patient's mouth. It is important to ensure suction is applied only to the mouth and pharynx. Putting the sucker near to the patient's larynx could induce laryngospasm. This is an airway emergency, and could result in the patient needing to be intubated, to be resolved.

When Andrzej returns to the recovery area, you note that he is able to maintain his own airway – and that there is no obvious sound as he takes breaths – indicating that his airway, at this stage, is clear. He has an oxygen mask on, with oxygen being delivered at 6 litres per minute. He also has a pulse oximeter in place, which currently shows oxygen saturation of 96 per cent.

- B – Breathing: Is the patient breathing normally? Can you see the patient's chest rise and fall gently? It is important, when counting respirations, that you do so for a full minute. Make sure that you cannot hear any wheezing, gurgling or snoring noises while the patient breathes. Watch, too, for any signs of effort being taken to breathe. For example, you may see a patient tense the strap muscles in their neck in an effort to breathe. If you suspect that the patient has an airway obstruction, you need to call the anaesthetist.

Sometimes the drugs used to paralyse a patient's muscles for major surgery may take longer than expected to wear off. The patient may be in a lot of pain, or their respiratory system may still be suppressed from anaesthetic agents or due to IV analgesics, such as morphine. Given that orthopaedic surgery is very painful, Andrzej will have been given and prescribed IV morphine for the initial stages of his recovery, so it will be important to continually review the impact that the IV morphine may be having on his respiration rate. Normally patients arriving in recovery after a general anaesthetic will be given oxygen to ensure that their oxygen saturation levels are maintained above 95 per cent. The administration of oxygen helps with the flushing of anaesthetic agents, particularly nitrous oxide, from the body.

On admission to recovery, Andrzej appears to be breathing normally – and his respiratory rate is currently at 14 bpm. His oxygen saturation is at 96 per cent. However, as he is prescribed bolus doses of IV morphine in the recovery area, this will need close monitoring. One of the most common reasons for a drop in respiratory rate in the PACU is the impact of IV opioid administration.

- C – Circulation and consciousness: The PACU nurse will take and record the patient's pulse and blood pressure every 5 minutes for the first 15 minutes initially, and continue to monitor every 15 minutes. The pulse needs to be assessed for rate, volume and rhythm (Liddle, 2013). Ideally, all observations should be recorded electronically. Pain and haemorrhage can both adversely affect a patient's cardiovascular system in the recovery unit. Given that Andrzej has already lost at least 1.5 litres of blood during surgery – and probably more, due to the nature of his trauma – these observations are really important. The PACU nurse will also look at a patient's colour, as bluish colouration of a patient's extremities can indicate problems with oxygenation levels. Many patients will have regained consciousness by the time they arrive in the recovery room; however, it is important to be vigilant, particularly after any IV analgesia has been given.

On admission, Andrzej's pulse is slightly elevated, at 85 bpm. His pulse and BP are monitored every 5 minutes for the first 15 minutes of his stay in the PACU and, as no issues arise, monitored every 15 minutes after this. His colour, including at his extremities, indicates that his perfusion status is good.

Andrzej has regained consciousness on return to the PACU – he is able to respond to requests to take a deep breath and to cough. However, he is still slightly drowsy. Hatfield (2014) gives useful insights into how Andrzej might perceive his recovery in the PACU. From his perspective, his first sense to return will be his hearing, meaning that loud voices or noises in the area may seem very frightening. Although challenging, it is important to try to keep noise levels in the PACU down. He may not be able to cope with bright lights, meaning that facilities for dimming lights may be necessary. His limbs may feel very heavy, and the pain he feels – particularly given that he has had orthopaedic surgery – may seem like the worst he has ever felt. He is also likely to feel disorientated for a while.

- D – Drugs, drips, dressings and drains: The anaesthetist should identify what drugs have been given to a patient during surgery. They will also ensure that they have written up prescriptions for analgesics, oxygen, anti-emetics and IV fluids that may be needed by the patient in the post-operative period. The anaesthetist should also ensure that all lines are flushed. This needs to be done to remove any residual anaesthetic drugs (AAGBI, 2013).

In the case of Andrzej, he will also need a prescription of antibiotics, as the nature of his injury makes him susceptible to post-operative infection. Some patients like Andrzej, if they have lost a lot of blood during surgery, will continue to have an IV infusion in place. It is important that the PACU nurse or nursing associate checks what IV fluids, and how much, have been given during surgery. It is important to check that IV lines are patent, that IV fluids are flowing freely at the correct rate, and that the IV cannula site is checked and re-secured and protected, if necessary (AAGBI, 2013).

It is important to check a patient's wound dressing when they come out of surgery. You may find that if there is some blood visible on the dressing, staff mark the extent of this, so they can gauge the amount of any subsequent bleeding. Although used less often, for some types of surgery, some patients may have a drain put in the wound site, and attached to a collection device, such as a suction bottle. This is in cases where it is important to drain any blood, pus or other fluid, to prevent it accumulating within the body.

Andrzej has had IV opioids administered during his operation, has been prescribed bolus doses of IV morphine and has had a drain inserted. There is a small amount of blood in Andrzej's drain, and no obvious bleeding through his dressing or on his sheets.

- E – Everything else (adapted E for post-operative care): Within the PACU setting it is helpful for the 'E' of the ABCDE assessment to consider 'everything else', which, it is acknowledged, differs from the other chapters. This is helpful, and shows the adaptability of the assessment approach. This could include: if the patient is a diabetic, do they need an insulin infusion? If they have had orthopaedic surgery, does the surgeon require them to have a splint in place to keep, for example, an operated leg in proper alignment?

One possible early post-operative complication of traumatic fractures, particularly of the shaft of the femur, is neurological damage from sharp bone ends (Tidy, 2021). In the case of Andrzej, this means that it will be important to carry out assessment of the neurovascular status of his right leg. This needs to be done every 30 minutes. It includes assessing the peripheral pulses in his leg, the colour and temperature of his leg, whether there is any numbness, tingling or swelling, and whether he can move his toes.

The other routine check that needs to be carried out – particularly in the case of someone who has suffered from a traumatic fractured femur – is to look for signs of fat emboli, which can sometimes be called Fat Emboli Syndrome (FES). Hatfield (2014) suggests that it is caused by fat from the bone marrow of the injured bone being released into the patient's blood stream. Once within the blood stream, the fat is broken down by enzymes. One of the products from this is free fatty acids. When these fatty acids reach the lungs, they are toxic to alveoli, and can set up an inflammatory reaction, which can result in pulmonary oedema. The circulating fat can also cause disseminated intravascular coagulation (DIC). Although this usually occurs 12–72 hours after injury, it may be seen in the PACU, particularly with patients who have been admitted the day before. Signs will be related to pulmonary oedema and include increasing breathlessness, increase in respiratory rate of over 20 bpm and a decrease in oxygen saturation. There may also be signs related to cerebral oedema, which can occur where there is damage to the capillaries in the brain, leading to leaking of fluid into the cerebral tissue. Signs can include increasing headaches, confusion and gradual loss of consciousness.

This condition is prevented by ensuring the broken limb is immobilised and stabilized as soon as possible after fracturing. Treatment may include the patient being ventilated in an intensive care unit for a few days.

On assessment, Andrzej currently displays none of the signs of FES.

Post-operative complications

Post-operative hypothermia

Most patients having surgery are at risk of post-operative hypothermia (Hatfield 2014). Some of the risk factors for post-operative hypothermia include extremes of age (very young or old), having surgery that takes more than three hours, burns patients or patients having surgery following major trauma. On admission to the PACU, Andrzej's temperature is 36 °C. The anaesthetist confirms that the perioperative team used a forced-air warming device (sometimes called a Bair Hugger™) when Andrzej was on the operating table.

If a patient is cold, they are likely to shiver in response to hypothermia. This increases the metabolic rate and oxygen consumption considerably, and can lead to hypoxia. Hypothermia can also lead to peripheral vasoconstriction, meaning that the heart has to work harder to ensure blood can continue to flow through constricted blood vessels, leading to possible myocardial ischemia, tissue hypoxia and lactic acidosis. Shivering can also contribute to increased levels of muscle pain (Hatfield 2014).

For Andrzej, his ability to maintain a normal body temperature will have been affected by several factors. This includes being anaesthetised for some time, and losing heat through having a large wound site, meaning body heat lost through evaporation, conduction, convection and radiation. Perioperative theatres are also usually kept cool, for the comfort of the surgical team, who operate wearing gloves and sterile gowns. If Andrzej continues to be hypothermic, this will affect his ability to metabolise and excrete drugs – which could prolong the effect of, for example, opioids. It may also delay his return to full consciousness. Hypothermia can also increase the chance of post-operative bleeding and increase the possibility of wound breakdown. It can also lead to a greater chance of post-operative infection, by supressing a patient's immune system.

It is important to check Andrzej's temperature carefully, using a tympanic membrane sensor or a rectal probe. Clinical thermometers should not be used, as they do not register low temperatures (Hatfield, 2014). Andrzej can be warmed gradually by applying an additional warm blanket. If a forced air warming device is available, then this can be used – however, these are not often available outside of the operating theatre. It may take Andrzej some time – up to 12 hours – for his temperature to come back to normal. However, applying a blanket should prevent his temperature dropping further. It will be important to continue to record his temperature, and to ensure that he continues to receive oxygen, to help his body cope with increased oxygen requirements if he shivers.

Pain

Waking up in pain in the PACU after anaesthesia can be extremely distressing for the patient. However, it is possible to control pain quickly in this setting, through the use of opioids, using titrated intravenous doses. This can be supplemented through the use of other methods of controlling pain, such as the use of Patient Controlled Analgesia (PCA). It is really important to control acute pain as quickly as possible – failure to do so effectively can result in a patient developing chronic pain.

The best way of treating acute pain in this setting is to ask patients about their pain – given that pain is a subjective experience, verbal reports, for patients who are conscious and able to understand what they are being asked to describe, are seen as a gold standard and commonly used in PACU. A variety of pain scales can be used to assess the acuity of pain (Luo and Min, 2017) and include:

- visual analog scale (VAS) – where a long line is drawn, with one end labelled no pain and the other end worst possible pain;
- numerical rating scale (NRS) – where patients are given a 10-point scale, with 1 meaning they have no pain, and 10 meaning they have the worst pain ever;
- verbal rating scale (VRS) – where patients describe their pain as mild, moderate, severe, very severe;
- Wong–Baker face pain rating scale – where patients point out a face that best represents the pain that they are feeling.

However, some authors suggest that given that many patients may not be able to give a verbal response in the PACU, due to the effects of anaesthesia and surgery, using scales or relying on verbal reports may not always be appropriate (Lewis et al., 2013). Once the PACU team assess the degree of pain, then it is important that sufficient analgesia is given as soon as possible to alleviate the pain.

Given that Andrzej has had an ORIF to fix a traumatic fracture to his femur, the PACU team should expect that he will experience severe pain. The anaesthetist gave IV morphine to Andrzej in the operating theatre, prior to him being transferred to the PACU. He has been prescribed IV morphine – this is usually prepared using 10mg morphine in a solution of 10ml saline, to give a strength of 1mg/ml.

As Andrzej regains consciousness, he becomes restless, and his pulse rate increases to 100 bpm. His blood pressure is raised slightly, to 125/80. His respiratory rate is 12 bpm and oxygen saturation is 95 per cent. The PACU nurse asks him about his pain level – he is able to respond that his pain feels severe. The PACU nurse gives a titrated dose of morphine – 2ml/IV. She waits three minutes before asking Andrzej how his pain feels now. He says that his pain still feels severe. She gives a further titrated dose of morphine – 2ml/IV. Three minutes later, she again asks Andrzej what level his pain is. He says that it is still bad, but not as severe. His respiratory rate is still 12 breaths per minute, and his BP has dropped slightly, to 120/80. She gives a further dose of morphine – but this time gives 1ml/IV. Three minutes later, Andrzej reports that his pain is more manageable. His pulse rate has reduced to 80 bpm. Another sign that Andrzej had enough opioids would be if he became drowsy but still rousable, or if his respiration rate dropped to between 8 and 10 breaths per minute (Hatfield, 2014).

Haemorrhage and hypovolaemia

You will have seen in Chapter 9 that Andrzej developed hypovolaemic shock, prior to coming to theatres for surgery. It is worth reviewing the signs, symptoms and treatment of hypovolaemic shock. Any patient coming for major surgery – particularly trauma surgery, will be at risk of bleeding and developing hypovolaemia. Young adults, who are otherwise healthy, can sustain a blood loss equating to about 30 per cent (1.5 litres) of their blood volume before this haemorrhage becomes life-threatening (Hatfield, 2014). It is worth noting that for some previously healthy adults, the ability of their body to compensate for blood loss means that their blood pressure may not initially drop in response to acute blood loss.

The most common cause of rapid blood loss in the PACU is related to haemostasis of the surgical site. As a patient recovers from anaesthesia, their blood pressure may rise sufficiently to loosen a surgical tie used to stop bleeding, or the rise causes a blood vessel to start to bleed. Given that Andrzej has a wound drain inserted, it is important to check this, and the area around the wound site and sheets, for external signs of bleeding. If you note more than 100mls of blood draining in 30 minutes, then call the surgeon.

For some patients, bleeding may not be visible or obvious – particularly following abdominal surgery or surgery on the femur or thoracic cavity. In these cases, a large amount of blood can collect in internal cavities – in excess of 1.5 litres – before swelling is evident. Signs may include a rising tachycardia (above 110 bpm), increasing respiratory rate, decreased urine output, and a deterioration in the patient's level of consciousness – including increasing levels of anxiety, agitation and confusion (Hatfield, 2014). If you suspect a patient is losing a lot of blood in the PACU, it is important to call for help immediately. Lay the patient flat if possible, raise their legs (if possible), continue to deliver 6/l per minute of oxygen, check for obvious signs of bleeding and, if possible, apply direct pressure on the area using a pad and, wearing gloves, continue to monitor pulse and blood pressure. You will also need to call the anaesthetist and surgeon. In some instances, a patient may require a blood transfusion. In other instances, they may need to be transferred back to theatre, so that the surgeon can deal with any internal bleeding directly.

Safe transfer to ward

Patients need to remain in the PACU until recovery staff are confident that it is safe to transfer them back to the ward area. If the PACU team have any doubt as to whether or not the patient meets the discharge criteria, then they need to call the anaesthetist, who must come to assess the patient. If the patient does not meet discharge criteria, they may need to be transferred to a HDU or ITU setting (AAGBI, 2013). Patients will be ready for transfer when:

- they are fully awake, responsive and able to maintain their own airway. Sometimes the recovery nurse will test this by asking a patient to lift and keep their head off the pillow for a short time;
- they are breathing normally and have adequate oxygenation levels;
- they are relatively pain-free and have adequate analgesia;
- their cardiovascular system is stable and their pulse and blood pressure are at levels nearer their normal pre-operative levels;
- their body temperature is within acceptable limits;
- there are no continuing surgical problems (for example, bleeding);
- the recovery staff can give clear instructions to the ward on post-operative care requirements (including oxygen, drugs and fluids).

After 90 minutes in the PACU, Andrzej is now fully awake and able to maintain his own airways. His observations are as below:

- heart rate (HR): 80 beats per minute (bpm);
- blood pressure (BP): 112/70 millimetres of mercury (mmHg);
- respiratory rate (RR): 12 breaths per minute (bpm);
- saturations (SpO2): 96%;
- Temperature (TEMP): 36.8 °C.

His pain is now well controlled, and his temperature is gradually rising. His wound site and drain do not show any additional blood. The anaesthetist has written up analgesics, antiemetics and IV fluids.

Given that Andrzej is at risk of developing a post-operative infection, he has been prescribed broad-spectrum antibiotics to be given IV.

It is helpful to consider your responsibilities if you were receiving Andrzej back into his ward; this is looked at in Activity 10.2.

Activity 10.2   Critical thinking

Looking at the transfer of Andrzej from A&E to the operating department (Chapter 9), and from the operating theatre to PACU (this chapter), how would you prepare Andrzej's bed and environment in order to safely care for him on his return to the ward.

An outline answer is provided at the end of this chapter.

Case study: Andrzej (continued)

Andrzej will now be transferred to the ward for post-operative care. Chapter 11 will continue Andrzej's care and the focus will be on his development of sepsis.

Chapter summary

This chapter has continued the case study of Andrzej commenced in the previous chapter. This chapter has focused on his immediate post-operative care following repair of his hip fracture, within the PACU, and included the priorities of care at this stage. The chapter has also reviewed common immediate post-operative problems including hypothermia, pain, haemorrhage and hypovolaemic shock. Safe patient transfers are key priorities throughout the patient's surgical journey, and these have been considered with supporting activities.

Activities: brief outline answers

Activity 10.1 Reflection

Some of the similarities in the set-up of areas to receive patients in both A&E and the PACU would include:

- oxygen and suction available and turned on, with additional equipment available to support a patient's airway – including a variety of airways and bag-valve-mask devices;
- monitoring devices available to monitor pulse, pulse oximetry, blood pressure;
- ready access to a range of IV fluids – and IV stands;
- ready access to a resuscitation trolley;
- ready access to a range of emergency drugs, analgesics and antibiotics;
- access to method of recording patient data and observations.

Some of the differences in the set-up of the PACU may include, for example, ensuring that each patient is cared for by a registered practitioner, with specific preparation to work in the PACU area. The environment in the PACU needs to be set up to ensure that lights and sounds are kept to a minimum, and that the team has access to additional warming devices, such as blankets or forced-air warming devices.

Activity 10.2 Critical thinking

When receiving a patient from the PACU, the ward bed needs to be set up to ensure:

- wall oxygen available – with face mask/oxygen administration system attached;
- suction device available and set up;
- monitoring available and checked – ideally non-invasive blood pressure monitoring and pulse oximetry, plus thermometer;
- drip stand, if needed;
- access to additional blankets if needed;
- charts (either electronic or paper) – to record patient observations.

Further reading

Hatfield, A. (2014) *The Complete Recovery Book* (5th Ed.). Oxford: Oxford University Press.

This is a very accessible and comprehensive guide to everything you might need to know about recovering a patient after surgery. You will find that some of the advice can be applied to caring for the surgical patient in the ward area too.

Armellino, D. (2017) Minimizing sources of airborne, aerosolized, and contact contaminants in the OR environment. *AORN Journal*, 106(6): 494–501.

This gives a detailed account of all possible sources of infection in the operating theatre, and advice on how to minimise these.

Gracia, M. (2016) Scrubbing up: My first experience as a student nurse in the operating theatre. *British Journal of Nursing*, 25(11): 621.

If you are offered the opportunity of scrubbing alongside a qualified member of staff, you might find it interesting to compare your experience with this student nurse. Most theatre staff will remember very well their first time scrubbing for a case.

Palmer, L. (2013) Anaesthesia 101: Everything you need to know. *Plastic Surgical Nursing*, 33(4): 164–71.

If you want to learn more about anaesthesia, this is a really useful starting point. It goes over the drugs used and key considerations.

Trigo, A. (2016) Monitoring during anaesthesia and recovery. *Nursing Management*, 23(8): 10.

This article provides a good overview of monitoring during anaesthesia and recovery.

Useful websites

www.who.int/patientsafety/safesurgery/ss_checklist/en/index.htm

World Health Organization (2008) Safe Surgery Saves Lives.

www.youtube.com/watch?v=CsNpfMldtyk

The WHO checklist

www.cochrane.org/search/site/surgical%20scrubbing

Useful resource of best evidence for healthcare practice. This particular page focuses on a specific area of perioperative practice.

https://twitter.com/CochraneUK

Twitter site of use for those who feel they do not have time to check up on latest findings.

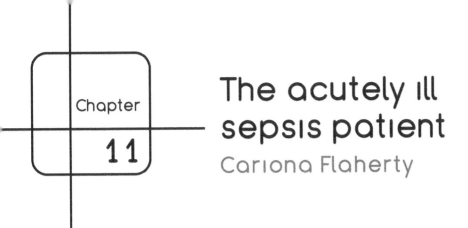

The acutely ill sepsis patient

Cariona Flaherty

Chapter aims

By the end of this chapter you should be able to:

- define what is meant by the term 'sepsis' and identify the associated risk factors;
- discuss the pathophysiology of sepsis;
- identify the common tools used to screen for sepsis, and how to assess an acutely ill sepsis patient;
- understand how to implement the 'Sepsis Six' when caring for a patient with sepsis;
- explain the role of human factors in sepsis.

Introduction

The UK Sepsis Trust (UKST) (2019, page 11), estimates that 'we see at least 200,000 cases of sepsis in the UK each year, with up to 52,000 deaths. The direct cost of sepsis on the NHS is estimated at £1.5 billion', and the cost of sepsis on our society is approximately £15.6 billion every year (UKST, 2019). Sepsis costs the NHS more than asthma, and 'claims more lives than lung cancer, and more than bowel, breast and prostate cancer combined' (UKST, 2019, page 9). The National Confidential Enquiry into Patient Outcome and Death (NCEPOD) (2015b) identified sepsis as the major cause of avoidable deaths. The survival of sepsis-induced hypotension is greater than '75% if recognised in a timely manner, but every hour's delay causes that figure to fall by over 7%' (NCEPOD, 2015b, page 5). The UKST (2019) highlighted that approximately 80,000 sepsis survivors will have one or more cognitive, psychological or physical life-changing after-effects. In 2016, Health Education England (HEE) (2016) made further changes to sepsis education and training for all healthcare professionals to ensure early recognition and rapid management of sepsis was implemented. However, the recognition and management of sepsis has become increasingly complex due to the ageing population, presentation of multiple comorbidities and the increased prevalence of antimicrobial resistance (Hird, 2020). This chapter will utilise the case study from Chapter 9 and 10, and focus on Andrzej's post-operative development of sepsis. The associated risk factors, and definition of sepsis and underpinning pathophysiology will be discussed. The screening tools used to identify suspected sepsis, and the framework for assessing an acutely ill sepsis patient will be explained. The management of sepsis will focus on implementation of the Sepsis Six, and the role of human factors in relation to sepsis will be addressed.

Case study: Andrzej, the acutely ill sepsis patient

Andrzej arrived in A&E following an RTA that sustained a right femur open compound fracture (see Chapter 9). Andrzej went to theatre and had an open reduction and internal fixation, with an estimated blood loss of 1 litre. Following surgery, Andrzej was transferred to the ward, where he developed a temperature, hypotension and decreased urine output. His observations were as follows:

(Continued)

(Continued)

- heart rate (HR): 110 beats per minute (bpm);
- blood pressure (BP): 90/50 millimetres of mercury (mmHg);
- respiratory rate (RR): >24 breaths per minute (bpm);
- saturations (SpO2): 94%;
- temperature (TEMP): 38.0°C.

Activity 11.1   Critical thinking

Go back to Chapter 2 and locate Figure 2.4 NEWS2 and Figure 2.5 NEWS2 Thresholds and triggers. Using this, calculate Andrzej's NEWS2 score, and identify whether there is a clinical risk and what response should be actioned for Andrzej.

An outline answer is given at the end of the chapter.

Sepsis definition and risk factors

There has been a number of definitions for sepsis, and variation of terms such as severe sepsis, sepsis shock, and organ dysfunction. The term severe sepsis was made redundant in 2016, and the terms now used across practices are sepsis and septic shock (Singer et al., 2016). The third international consensus definition for sepsis and septic shock (Sepsis-3) was updated in 2016 to 'sepsis is life-threatening organ dysfunction caused by dysregulated host response to infection (Singer et al., 2016, page 2). Septic shock is defined as 'a subset of sepsis, in which particularly profound circulatory, cellular, and metabolic abnormalities are associated with a greater risk of mortality than with sepsis alone' (Singer et al., 2016, page 2). The definitions for sepsis and septic

Consider that people in the following groups are at higher risk of developing sepsis	• the very young (under 1) and older people (over 75) • people who have impaired immune systems (people being treated for cancer) • people who have impaired immune function (diabetes, post splenectomy, sickle cell disease) • people taking long-term steroids • post-surgery (in the past 6 weeks) • people taking immunosuppressants • people with any breach in skin integrity • people with indwelling lines or catheters • people who misuse IV drugs
Consider women who are pregnant, have given birth or had termination of pregnancy or miscarriage in the past six weeks.	• In particular those who have: • impaired immune systems • diabetes or gestational diabetes • needed invasive procedures (caesarean section) • prolonged ruptured membrane (amniotic sac) • been in contact with group A streptococcal infection (scarlet fever) • vaginal bleeding or offensive discharge

Figure 11.1   Risk factors for sepsis in adults (adapted from NICE, 2016c, pages 7 and 8)

shock were given international consensus to reduce the potential for discrepancies in reporting, and to ensure greater consistency in early recognition and timely treatment (Singer et al., 2016). The first step to support you as an NA in identifying sepsis is to understand the risk factors. The National Institute for Health and Care Excellence (NICE) (2016c) identified risk factors for sepsis (see Figure 11.1).

Activity 11.2   Critical thinking

Read Andrzej's case study from Chapter 9, 10 and this chapter, and using the table in Figure 11.1, identify why Andrzej might be at risk of sepsis.
An outline answer is given at the end of the chapter.

Sepsis pathophysiology

Understanding the risk factors for sepsis is imperative to ensure early recognition of sepsis. It is also as important that you in your role as an NA understand sepsis pathophysiology so that you can provide justification for escalation of timely care and management. Hird (2020) identify that the pathophysiology of sepsis is complex and not fully understood. However, what is known is that sepsis is a syndrome that involves physiological, pathological and biochemical abnormalities all in response to infection caused by bacteria, fungi, viruses or parasites (Hird, 2020). The pathophysiology of sepsis presents itself as follows:

Gram-positive (Staphylococcus), gram-negative (E. coli) and fungal pathogens are most commonly noted in sepsis. The bacteria cell wall releases endotoxins (gram-positive cells) and exotoxins (gram-negative cells) that engage with macrophages

The pro-inflammatory response is activated by a number of cells within the immune system (white blood cells (WBC), macrophages, neutrophils and lymphocytes)

This leads to the release of cytokines (pro-inflammatory cytokines)

Pro-inflammatory cytokines act to kill microorganisms, activate the clotting cascade and WBC recruitment

Pro-inflammatory cytokines compromise the tight junctions between endothelial cells within blood vessels

This leads to leaky blood vessels and increased vascular permeability

Protein-rich fluid leaks from the intravascular compartment into extravascular interstitial spaces

This leads to increased fluid in the interstitial fluid, causing oedema

In sepsis the pro-inflammatory cytokine response can become dysregulated, and this leads to a loss of intravascular volume and hypovolaemia

The pro-inflammatory cytokine response is normally regulated by the release of anti-inflammatory cytokines

When there is an imbalance between the pro-inflammatory cytokines and the anti-inflammatory cytokines; this leads to sepsis

In sepsis there is also a dysregulation in the clotting cascade caused by an imbalance between pro-coagulant and anti-coagulant factors

This results in a condition known as disseminated intravascular coagulation (DIC) leading to multiple blood clots or uncontrolled bleeding

(Adapted from Cook et al. (2019); Hird, 2020)

The pathophysiology of sepsis is complex and it lends itself to the imbalance of a number of systems, which can result in mortality if not identified in a timely manner and managed appropriately.

Sepsis screening tool prehospital

The UKST has produce a sepsis screening tool prehospital (see Figure 11.2) that identifies red flags for possible sepsis (UKST, 2019). This tool should be implemented if a patient looks unwell or has a NEWS2 of 5 or above. Utilising this tool (Figure 11.2) ensures the timely handover of patients and communication of potential sepsis diagnosis. As an NA it is important for you to have awareness of the sepsis screening tool prehospital so that patients care can be escalated quickly and appropriately.

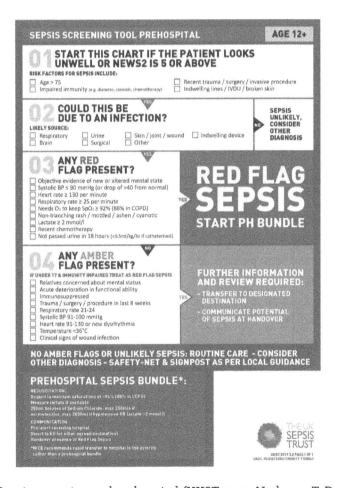

Figure 11.2 Sepsis screening tool prehospital (UKST, 2019; Nutbeam, T, Daniels, R on behalf of the UK Sepsis Trust, available at: sepsistrust.org/professional-resources/our-nice-clinical-tools/, accessed 16 August 2022)

Screening for sepsis

To complement the above prehospital screen tool, NICE (2017c) produced a risk stratification tool to support the assessment and recognition of suspected sepsis (please refer to the useful websites section at the end of this chapter). This places patients into high, moderate or low risk and is used widely within the NHS to support healthcare professionals with identifying suspected sepsis. Alongside the use of this tool, the NEWS2 remains pivotal in the identification of patients who are at risk of deteriorating. If you have not read Chapter 2, it would be good at this stage to pause, and refer to Chapter 2 for further information of the NEWS2. NICE's risk stratification tool also highlights how to manage patients who have identified as high, medium or low risk. This will be referred to later in the chapter when addressing the management of sepsis.

Within intensive care clinicians use the Sequential Organ Failure Assessment (SOFA). A SOFA looks at organ dysfunction associated with sepsis, and a score of 2 points or more denotes an increase in mortality of greater than 10 per cent (Singer et al., 2016). Outside of intensive care settings, the Quick Sequential Organ Failure Assessment (qSOFA) is used to rapidly identify patients with sepsis at risk of poor outcomes. qSOFA sepsis looks at the following scoring:

- respiratory rate of 22/min or greater (+1 Point);
- altered mentation (+1 Point);
- systolic BP </= 100 mmHg (+1 point).

A qSOFA score of 2 points or more is associated with poor patient outcomes (Singer et al., 2016). As an NA you may work in an intensive care setting or have placements there during your training. It is important that you become familiar with the scoring tools used within and outside of intensive care units.

Activity 11.3   Critical thinking

Reflecting on Andrzej's observations, what would Andrzej's qSOFA score be?
An outline answer is given at the end of the chapter.

Assessing the acutely ill sepsis patient

Having identified a patient at risk of sepsis, the next step is to carry out a full comprehensive patient assessment. As previously discussed throughout this book, the ABCDE assessment framework should be utilised to assess the acutely ill patient. Chapter 2 provides an in-depth ABCDE assessment which follows RCUK (2021b). This section will provide a brief overview of Andrzej's ABCDE assessment, utilising the information from Chapters 9, 10 and this chapter.

ABCDE assessment of Andrzej

| **First steps** | • personal safety; |
| | • ask Andrzej how he is. |

Airway	•	Andrzej has not reported signs of airway obstruction post-operatively and arrived on the ward maintaining his own airway.
Breathing	•	normal breath sound r;
	•	respiratory rate (RR): >24 bpm;
	•	oxygen saturations level (SpO2): 94%;
	•	listen to Andrzej's breath sounds, and check for equal and bilateral rise and fall of the chest wall;
	•	percuss and auscultate Andrzej's chest (if trained to do so).
Circulation	•	look at the colour of Andrzej's hands and fingers;
	•	temp 38.0 °C;
	•	measure Andrzej's capillary refill time;
	•	assess the state of Andrzej's veins and urine output status;
	•	heart rate (HR): 110 bpm;
	•	blood pressure (BP): 100/50 mmHg;
	•	temperature (TEMP): 38.0 °C;
	•	ascertain IV access status;
	•	complete an ECG.
Disability	•	GCS 15/15, sleepy post-operatively;
	•	examine Andrzej's pupil size, and measure blood glucose level.
Exposure	•	post-surgical wound drain, minimal drainage;
	•	wound dressing oozing.

NICE (2017d, page 8) stated that everyone with suspected sepsis should have the following assessed and examined:

- temperature;
- heart rate;
- respiratory rate;
- level of consciousness;
- oxygen saturations;
- mottled skin appearance;
- cyanosis of the skin, lips or tongue;
- signs of a non-blanching rash;
- skin integrity;
- any form of rash that could indicate infection.

NICE (2017d, page 9) highlighted that the symptoms of sepsis include (but are not limited to) the following:

- high or low temperature;
- increased HR or RR;
- dizzy, faint, loss of conscious;
- confusion;
- diarrhoea, nausea or vomiting;
- slurred speech;
- severe muscle pain;
- breathlessness;
- reduced urine output;
- cold, clammy, pale or mottled skin.

Reflecting on Andrzej's ABCDE assessment, and NICE (2017c, 2017d), list the symptoms that are most concerning.

An outline answer is given at the end of the chapter.

Case study: Andrzej (continued)

Andrzej appears to have deteriorated further, his urine output has reduced, and he appears confused and disorientated. He appears cold and clammy and his observations are as follows:

- heart rate (HR): 120 beats per minute (bpm);
- blood pressure (BP): 89/50 millimetres of mercury (mmHg);
- respiratory rate (RR): >24 breaths per minute (bpm);
- saturations (SpO2): 92%;
- temperature (TEMP): 38.5 °C.

Management of sepsis

Andrzej's NEWS2 score is now 10, and as per the NEWS trigger system this required an urgent response. The critical care team arrived on the ward, and started Andrzej's on the Sepsis Six protocol for suspected sepsis, with the origin or infection likely being from his open compound fracture. Although the care of Andrzej at this point has been escalated, your role as an NA will be to support the registered nurses with providing care for Andrzej; that is within your remit as an NA. In order to support the nurses, you must understand what the Sepsis Six is. The Sepsis Six was introduced in 2006 by the UKST, with a view to streamlining the management of sepsis. Although the Sepsis Six has undergone minor changes since it was first introduced, it remains fundamental in the treatment of sepsis, and is now used across more than 30 countries (Dean, 2021). The founder and clinical director of the UKST stated that 'the success of the Sepsis Six is that it is rooted in evidence but it is not heavily academic. It is a simple tool (Dean, 2021, page 53). The aforementioned NICE (2017c) 'Risk Stratification Tool: people aged 18 and over in hospital' echoes the Sepsis Six, but provides in-depth information on clinical values.

The UKST (2020) outlines the Sepsis Six and actions as follows:

1. Ensure senior clinician attends.
2. Oxygen ff required: start O2 if saturations < 92% and aim for O2 saturations of 94-98%. If at risk of hypercapnia (high CO2) aim for O2 saturations 88–92%.
3. Obtain IV access, take bloods: blood culture, blood glucose, lactate, full blood count (FBC), urea and electrolytes (U&Es), c-reactive protein (CRP) and clotting. Lumbar puncture as indicated.
4. Give IV antibiotics: maximum dose broad spectrum therapy.
5. Give IV fluids: give fluid bolus of 20ml/kg if age <16, 500mls if 16+.
6. Monitor: Use NEWS2, urine output, repeat lactate at least once per hour if initial lactate was elevated.

All of the above should be completed within one hour.

Figure 11.3 Further detailed information on the UKST sepsis screening tool – Sepsis Six (UKST, 2019; Nutbeam, T, Daniels, R on behalf of the UK Sepsis Trust, available at: sepsistrust.org/professional-resources/our-nice-clinical-tools/ (accessed: 16 August 2022)

Case study: Andrzej (continued)

Following transfer to critical care, Andrzej was seen again by a senior clinician. He was commenced on O2 60 per cent initially via a face mask to aim for oxygen saturations > 94 per cent. A large IV cannula was inserted, and blood cultures, blood glucose levels, lactate, FBC, U&Es, CRP and clotting were completed. He was started on broad spectrum IV antibiotics, and IV fluids initial doses of 500mls, aiming for a systolic BP > 100 mmHg. Andrzej was on hourly observations, urine output and lactate monitoring. The senior clinician explained to Andrzej that he was being treated for sepsis.

Human factors in sepsis

NCEPOD (2015b, page 18) stated that 'early recognition and management of sepsis leads to a reduction in morbidity and mortality, and administration of an effective antimicrobial within the first hour of hypotension has been associated with a survival rate of 79.9%'. Wentowski, Ingles and Nielsen (2021) echo this, highlighting that the implementation of the 1-hour Bundle Sepsis Six is essential for improving patient outcomes. However, despite advances in sepsis recognition and management, the mortality rates for sepsis remain high. The UKST (2019) discussed the role that human factors have in recognising and managing patients with sepsis. The World Health Organisation (WHO) (2016) identified human factors as physical, cognitive and organisational, all of which influence our behaviour. Having awareness of how human factors can influence patient safety is imperative. For example, in healthcare we work long shifts, deal with multiple tasks and often have staff shortages, all of which if not supported and managed carefully can lead to work burnout, mistakes and ultimately the compromising of patient safety. The UKST (2019, page 107) further explains that human factors encompass 'non-technical skills such as leadership, decision-making and performance', all of which directly affect how people work and behave. Understanding how the environment we work in, and the people we work with, can affect our behaviour and lead to human errors is vital. Therefore, training on human factors should form part of all sepsis-related training. The UKST (2019, page 108) stated that 'effective leadership is vital alongside education and training to raise awareness around the importance of human factors in healthcare and promote a safety culture in the effective management of sepsis'.

Activity 11.5 Reflection

To further support your understanding of human factors, please watch the video titled 'Just a routine operation' on YouTube (see the section on useful websites at the end of this chapter). This video highlights how human factors contributed to the death of a woman admitted to hospital for a routine operation. This training video highlighted how the lack of training in relation to human factors led to the breakdown in leadership, communication and teamwork.

As this activity is based on your own reflection, no outline answer is given at the end of the chapter.

Sepsis training should include awareness of human factors, as this is a fundamental aspect of patient care. HEE (2016) published a report on 'Getting it right: The current state of sepsis education and training for healthcare staff across England'. Within this report HEE made a number of recommendations to improve sepsis education and training, such as:

- updating all training in line with the NICE Sepsis Guidelines (2017d);
- all healthcare staff are to be trained and updated on sepsis;
- consider introducing 'Sepsis Champions';
- monitoring the effects of training;
- online training to include interactive elements;
- using clinical incidence related to sepsis where possible as learning opportunities.

WHO (2018) also produced an easy-to-follow guide outlining strategies to support the prevention of sepsis (see the useful websites section at the end of this chapter for the weblink). Education and training are fundamental in developing awareness of sepsis, early recognition and within the hour commencement of treatment.

Case study: Andrzej (continued)

Andrzej was started on treatment early, and as such began to show signs of improvement within the first 24 hours. Andrzej was admitted to A&E in Chapter 9 following an RTA with a right femur open compound fracture. Andrzej went to theatre in Chapter 10, and had an open reduction and internal fixation. From reading this chapter and in particular the NICE (2016c) risk factors for sepsis, you should now be able to identify that having an open wound alone puts Andrzej at risk of developing sepsis. This risk increased because Andrzej then had surgery.

Andrzej's sepsis was identified early and managed, and because of this, Andrzej was discharged from hospital with no long-term life-limiting side effects.

Chapter summary

This chapter started by defining sepsis and highlighting the associated risk factors. The underpinning pathophysiology was addressed, and the sepsis prehospital screening tool was discussed. Screening for sepsis including information on the sepsis risk stratification tool, NEWS2, SOFA and qSOFA. Following this the ABCDE assessment was utilised to complete a comprehensive patient assessment. The management of sepsis utilised the Sepsis Six, and the importance of implementing this within one hour was discussed. A number of activities and a case study were included to support your learning. This chapter finalised with an overview of the importance of human factors, and the common approaches used to prevent sepsis were addressed.

Activities: brief outline answers

Activity 11.1 Critical thinking

Andrzej's NEWS2 score = 7
Action based on the threshold and triggers = urgent or emergency response required, the response team must also include staff with critical care skills, including airway management.

Activity 11.2 Critical thinking

Andrzej would be at risk because he had an open compound fracture, recent surgery, and invasive lines (IV cannula, and catheter).

Activity 11.3 Critical thinking

Andrzej's qSOFA score = +2

Activity 11.4 Reflection

- \>24 breaths per minute (bpm);
- temperature 38.0°C;
- HR 110 beats per minute.

Useful websites

https://sepsistrust.org/about/about-sepsis/

The UK Sepsis Trust website provides an excellent number of resources to further support learning about sepsis.

www.sepsis.org/

Sepsis Alliance is an excellent website that provides support and guidance for those affected by sepsis.

www.who.int/news-room/fact-sheets/detail/sepsis

You can find useful easy to read information on sepsis via this World Health Organization website.

https://chfg.org/

Clinical Human Factors Group website provides comprehensive information and training that will further your understanding on human factors.

www.nice.org.uk/guidance/ng51/resources/algorithms-and-risk-stratification-tables-compiled-version-2551488301

This website provides information on risk stratification tools for people aged 18 and over in hospital.

https://youtu.be/JzlvgtPIof4

Laerdal Medical (2011) Just a Routine Operation (YouTube) - on the importance of human factors.

References

Adam, S., Osborne, S. and Welch, J. (2017) *Critical Care Nursing: Science and Practice* (3rd edn). Oxford: Oxford University Press.

Ahmed, A. and Stanley, A.J. (2012) Acute upper gastrointestinal bleeding in the elderly: Aetiology, diagnosis and treatment. *Drugs & Aging*, 29(12): 933–40.

Alexiou, A. and Rau, C. (2022) Shock. *BMJ Best Practice*. Available at: https://bestpractice.bmj.com/topics/en-gb/3000121 (accessed 4 April 2022).

Alzoubaidi, D. Lovat, L.B. and Haidry, R. (2019). Management of non-variceal upper gastrointestinal bleeding: Where are we in 2018?. *Frontline Gastroenterology*, 10(1): 35–42.

Ashelford, S., Raynsford, J. and Taylor, V. (2019) *Pathophysiology and Pharmacology in Nursing* (2nd edn.). London: SAGE.

Association of Anaesthetists of Great Britain and Ireland (2013) Immediate post-anaesthesia recovery 2013. *Anaesthesia*, 68(3): 288–97.

Barclay, J. and Jones, D. (2018) Stroke 4: Immediate treatment of acute stroke and TIA. *Nursing Times*, 114(2): 51–4.

Barrett, D., Gretton, M. and Quinn, T. (2006) *Cardiac Care: An Introduction for Healthcare Professionals*. Chichester: Wiley.

Bersten, A. and Soni, N. (2013) *Oh's Intensive Care Manual (Seventh Edition)*. Available at: https://doi.org/10.1016/B978-0-7020-4762-6.00126-0 (accessed 22nd September 2022).

Boore, J., Cook, N. and Shepherd, A. (2016) *Essentials of Anatomy and Physiology for Nursing Practice*. London: SAGE.

British Heart Foundation (2018) *Cardiac Rehab Saves Lives*. Available at: www.bhf.org.uk/for-professionals/healthcare-professionals/blog/2018/cardiac-rehab-saves-lives-so-why-do-half-of-patients-fail-to-show-up (accessed 24 January 2021).

British Heart Foundation (2022) *UK Factsheet*. Available at: www.bhf.org.uk/-/media/files/research/heart-statistics/bhf-cvd-statistics-england-factsheet.pdf?la=en (accessed 15 September 2022).

British National Formulary (BNF) (2021a) *Asthma, Acute*. Available at: https://bnf.nice.org.uk/treatment-summary/asthma-acute.html (accessed 19 November 2021).

British National Formulary (BNF) (2021b) *Alteplase*. Available at: https://bnf.nice.org.uk/drug/alteplase.html (accessed 28 November 2021).

British National Formulary (BNF) (2022a) *Drugs Affecting the Renin Angiotensin System*. Available at: https://bnf.nice.org.uk/treatment-summary/drugs-affecting-the-renin-angiotensin-system.html

British National Formulary (BNF) (2022b) *Non-steroidal Anti-inflammatory Drugs*. Available at: https://bnf.nice.org.uk/treatment-summary/non-steroidal-anti-inflammatory-drugs.html

References

British National Formula (2022c) *Metformin Hydrochloride.* Available at: https://bnf.nice.org.uk/drugs/metformin-hydrochloride/ (accessed 18 September 2022).

British Thoracic Society (BTS) (2019) *SIGN 158 British Guideline on the Management of Asthma.* Available at: www.brit-thoracic.org.uk/quality-improvement/guidelines/asthma/ (accessed 10 November 2021).

Castellanos, E.R., Seron, P., Gisbert, J.P. and Bonfill Cosp, X. (2012) Endoscopic injection of cyanoacrylate glue versus other endoscopic procedures for acute bleeding gastric varices in patients with portal hypertension. *Cochrane Database of Systematic Reviews*, 10. Art. No.: CD010180. Available at: www.cochranelibrary.com/cdsr/doi/10.1002/14651858.CD010180/full (accessed 19 January 2022).

Chapman, W., Siau, K., Thomas, F., Ernest, S., Begum, S., Iqbal, T. and Bhala, N. (2019) Acute upper gastrointestinal bleeding: A guide for nurses. PubMed.gov. Available at: https://pubmed.ncbi.nlm.nih.gov/30620657/ (accessed 14 March 2022).

Clarke, D. and Beaumont, P. (2016) Acute stroke. In Clarke, D. and Ketchell, A. (eds), *Nursing the Acutely Ill Adult: Priorities in Assessment and Management* (pp. 112–39). Basingstoke: Palgrave Macmillan.

Cook, N., Shepherd, A., Boore, J. and Dunleavy, S. (2019) *Essentials of Pathophysiology for Nursing Practice.* London: SAGE.

Cook, N., Shepherd, A. and Boore, J. (2021a) *Essentials of Anatomy and Physiology for Nursing Practice* (2nd edn). London: SAGE.

Cook, N., Shepherd, A., Dunleavy, S. and McCauley, C. (2021b) *Essentials of Pathophysiology for Nursing Practice* (2nd edn). London: SAGE.

Dean, E. (2021) The Sepsis Six toll: Steps to save a life. *Nursing Standard*, 36(10): 51–4.

Department of Health (2007) *National Stroke Strategy.* Available at: https://nsnf.org.uk/assets/documents/dh_081059.pdf (accessed 28 November 2021).

Department of Health (2009) *Stroke: Act F.A.S.T. Awareness Campaign.* Available at: http://webarchive.nationalarchives.gov.uk/20130107105354/http://www.dh.gov.uk/en/Publicationsandstatistics/Publications/PublicationsPolicyAndGuidance/DH_094239 (accessed 28 November 2021).

Desai, D., Mehta, D,. Mathias, P,. Menon, G. and Schubart, U.K. (2018) Health care utilization and burden of diabetic ketoacidosis in the U.S. over the past decade: A nationwide analysis. *Diabetes Care*, 41: 1631–8.

Diabetes UK (2021) *Blood Sugar Ranges.* Available at: www.diabetes.co.uk/diabetes_care/blood-sugar-level-ranges.html (accessed 14 January 2022).

DiGregorio, A.M. and Alvey, H. (2021) *Gastrointestinal Bleeding.* Available at: www.ncbi.nlm.nih.gov/books/NBK537291/ (accessed 14 March 2022).

Dougherty, L. and Lister, S. (2015) *The Royal Marsden Hospital Manual of Clinical Procedures* (9th edn). Hoboken, NJ: Wiley.

Dutton, H. and Finch, J. (2018) *Acute and Critical Care Nursing at a Glance.* Oxford: Wiley Blackwell.

Farsani, S.F., Brodovicz, K., Soleymanlou, N., Marquard, J., Wissinger, E. and Maiese, B.A. (2017) Incidence and prevalence of diabetic ketoacidosis (DKA) among adults with type 1 diabetes mellitus (T1D): A systematic literature review. *British Medical Journal*, 7: e016587.

Gibb, F.W., Teoh, W.L., Graham, J. and Lockman, K.A. (2016) Risk of death following admission to a UK hospital with diabetic ketoacidosis. *Diabetologia*, 59: 2082–7.

Global Initiative for Asthma (GINA) (2019) *Global Strategy for Asthma Management and Prevention.* Available at: https://ginasthma.org/wp-content/uploads/2019/06/GINA-2019-main-report-June-2019-wms.pdf (accessed 19 November 2021).

Goulden, I. and Clarke, D. (2016) Traumatic brain injury. In Clarke, D. and Ketchell, A. (eds), *Nursing the Acutely Ill Adult: Priorities in Assessment and Management* (pp. 88–111). Basingstoke: Palgrave Macmillan.

Hamdy, O. (2021) Diabetic Ketoacidosis (DKA). *Medscape.* Available at: https://emedicine.medscape.com/article/118361-overview (accessed 14 January 2022).

Hatfield, A. (2014) *The Complete Recovery Book* (5th edn). Oxford: Oxford University Press.

Health Education England (2015) *Raising the Bar Shape of Caring: A Review of the Future Education of Registered Nurses and Care Assistants.* Available at: www.hee.nhs.uk/sites/default/files/documents/2348-Shape-of-caring-review-FINAL.pdf (accessed October 18 2012).

Health Education England (2016) *Getting It Right: The Current State of Sepsis Education and Training for Healthcare Staff across England.* Available at: www.hee.nhs.uk/sites/default/files/documents/Getting%20it%20right%20The%20current%20state%20of%20sepsis%20education%20and%20training%20for%20healthcare%20staff%20across%20England.pdf (accessed 5 May 2022).

Health Education England (2017) *Nursing Associate Curriculum Framework.* Available at: www.hee.nhs.uk/sites/default/files/documents/Nursing%20Associate%20Curriculum%20Framework%20Feb2017_0.pdf (accessed October 14 2021).

Health Education England (2021) *Cardiovascular Disease.* Available at: www.hee.nhs.uk/our-work/population-health/cardiovascular-disease (accessed: 24 november 2021).

Hird, C. (2020) Early diagnosis and effective management of sepsis. *Nursing Standard*, 35: 59–66.

Hulse, C. and Davies, A. (2015) Acute kidney injury: Prevention and recognition. *Nursing Times*, 111(30/31): 12–15.

Hunt, B.J. Allard, S., Keeling, D., Norfolk, D., Stanworth, S.J. and Pendry, K. (2015) A practical guideline for the haematological management of major haemorrhage. *British Journal of Haematology*, 170(6): 788–803.

Institute for Innovation & Improvement (2017) *Safer Care: Situation, Background, Assessment & Recommendation.* Available at: www.england.nhs.uk/improvement-hub/wp-content/uploads/sites/44/2017/11/SBAR-Implementation-and-Training-Guide.pdf (accessed 6 December 2021).

Jevon, P. (2007) *Treating the Critical Care Patient.* Oxford: Blackwell.

Joint British Diabetes Societies for Inpatient Care (2021) *The Management of Diabetic Ketoacidosis in Adults.* Available at: www.diabetes.org.uk/professionals/position-statements-reports/specialist-care-for-children-and-adults-and-complications/the-management-of-diabetic-ketoacidosis-in-adults (accessed 15 September 2022).

Jones, K. and Steggall, M. (2020) Nursing patients with urinary disorders. In Peate, I. (ed.), *Nursing Practice: Hospital and Home.* London: Elsevier.

Kahi, C.J. Jensen, D.M. Sung, J.J. Bleau, B.L. Jung, H.K. Eckert, G. and Imperiale, T.F. (2005) Endoscopic therapy versus medical therapy for bleeding peptic ulcer with adherent clot: A meta-analysis. *Gastroenterology*, 129(3): 855–62.

References

Kanagasundaram, S., Ashley, C., Bhojani, S., Caldwell, A., Ellam, T., Kaur, A., Milford, D., Mulgrew, C. and Ostermann, M. (2019) *Clinical Practice Guideline: Acute Kidney Injury (AKI)*. The Renal Association. Available at: https://ukkidney.org/sites/renal.org/files/FINAL-AKI-Guideline.pdf

Kaufman, G. (2011) Asthma: Pathophysiology, diagnosis, and management. *Nursing Standard*, 26(5): 48–56.

Laerdal Medical (2011) *Just a Routine Operation*. Available at: https://youtu.be/JzlvgtPIof4 (accessed 5 May 2022).

Lewis, E., Craig, M. and Johnson, L. (2013) Use of the pain assessment behavioral scale (PABS) in PACU. *Journal of Perianesthesia Nursing*, 28(3): e47–8.

Liddle, C. (2013) Postoperative care 1: Principles of monitoring postoperative patients. *Nursing Times*, 109: 22, 24–6.

Loftus, N. and Smith, D. (2018) Investigation wards nurses' responses to deteriorating patients. *Nursing Standard*, 34(3): 76–82.

Luo, J. and Min, S. (2017) Postoperative pain management in the postanesthesia care unit: An update. *Journal of Pain Research*, 10: 2687–98.

Malecki-Ketchell, A. (2016) Coronary syndrome. In Clarke, D. and Malecki-Ketchell, A. (eds), *Nursing the Acutely Ill Adult* (pp. 140–84). London: Bloomsbury.

Marcovitch, H. (2005) *Black's Medical Dictionary*. London: Black.

Mason, M.C., Griggs, R.K., Withecombe, R., Xing, E.Y., Sandberg, C. and Molyneux, M.K. (2018) Improvement in staff compliance with a safety standard checklist in endoscopy in a tertiary centre. *BMJ Open Quality*, 7(3), e000294. Available at: https://doi.org/10.1136/bmjoq-2017-000294 (accessed 3 November 2021).

Massey, D., Aitken, L. and Chaboyer, W. (2008) What factors influence suboptimal ward care in the acutely ill ward patient? *Australian Critical Care*, 21(3): 127–40.

McCarty, T.R. and Njei, B. (2016). Self-expanding metal stents for acute refractory esophageal variceal bleeding: A systematic review and meta-analysis. *Digestive Endoscopy: Official Journal of the Japan Gastroenterological Endoscopy Society*, 28(5): 539–47.

McLafferty, E., Johnstone, C., Hendry, C. and Farley, A. (2013) Respiratory system part 1: pulmonary ventilation. *Nursing Standard*, 27(23): 35–42.

McRae, R. (2006) *Pocketbook of Orthopaedics and Fractures*. Edinburgh: Churchill Livingstone Elsevier.

Miraflor, E., Yeung, L., Strumwasser, A.T. and Victorino, G. (2012) *Emergency Uncrossmatched Transfusion Effect on Blood Type Alloantibodies*. PubMed.gov. Available at: https://pubmed.ncbi.nlm.nih.gov/22310115/ (accessed 4 April 2022).

Nagalingam, K. (2019) Urinary disorders. In Peate, I. (ed.) *Learning to Care: The Nursing Associate*. London: Elsevier.

National Confidential Enquiry into Patient Outcomes and Deaths (NCEPOD) (2015a). *Gastrointestinal Haemorrhage: Time to Get Control?* Available at: www.ncepod.org.uk/2015gih.html (accessed 14 March 2022).

National Confidential Enquiry into Patient Outcomes and Deaths (NCEPOD) (2015b) *Just Say Sepsis! A Review of the Process of Care Received by Patients with Sepsis*. Available at: www.ncepod.org.uk/2015report2/downloads/JustSaySepsis_FullReport.pdf (accessed 5 May 2022).

National Health Service Clinical Advisory Group on Trauma (2010) *Regional Networks for Major Trauma*. Available at: www.kcl.ac.uk/cicelysaunders/about/rehabilitation/The-NHS-Clinical-Advisory-Group-Report-on-Regional-Networks-for-Major-Trauma-(2010).pdf (accessed 16 September 2022).

National Health Service England (2019) *The NHS Long Term Plan*. Available at: www.longtermplan.nhs.uk/ (accessed 24 November 2021).

National Health Service England (2020) *Use of PPE*. Available at: www.england.nhs.uk/coronavirus/publication/guidance-supply-use-of-ppe/ (accessed 16 December 2021).

National Health Service England (2021a) *Diabetic Ketoacidosis*. Available at: www.nhs.uk/conditions/diabetic-ketoacidosis/ (accessed 24 March 2021).

National Health Service England (2021b) *National Stroke Services Model Integrated Stroke Delivery Networks*. Available at: www.england.nhs.uk/wp-content/uploads/2021/05/national-stroke-service-model-integrated-stroke-delivery-networks-may-2021.pdf (accessed 28 November 2021).

National Health Service England (2021c) *SBAR Communication Tool: Situation, Background, Assessment, Recommendation*. Available at: www.england.nhs.uk/wp-content/uploads/2021/03/qsir-sbar-communication-tool.pdf (accessed 28 March 2022).

National Institute for Health and Care Excellence (NICE) (2007) *Acutely Ill Patients in Hospital: Recognition of and Response to Acute Illness in Adults in Hospital*. Available at: www.nice.org.uk/guidance/cg50/evidence/full-guideline-195219037 (accessed 28 March 2022).

National Institute for Health and Care Excellence (NICE) (2014) *Acute Coronary Syndromes (Including Myocardial Infarction)*. Available at: www.nice.org.uk/guidance/qs68/documents/acute-coronary-syndromes-including-myocardial-infarction-briefing-paper2 (accessed 24 November 2021).

National Institute for Health and Care Excellence (NICE) (2016a) *Acute Upper Gastrointestinal Bleeding in over 16s: Management*. Clinical Guideline [CG141]. Available at: www.nice.org.uk/guidance/cg141 (accessed 1 November 2021).

National Institute for Health and Care Excellence (2016b) *Management of Haemorrhage in Pre-hospital and Hospital Settings*. Available at: www.nice.org.uk/guidance/NG39/chapter/Recommendations#management-of-haemorrhage-in-prehospital-and-hospital-settings (accessed 4 April 2022).

National Institute for Health and Care Excellence (NICE) (2016c) *Sepsis: Recognition, Diagnosis and Early Management*. Available at: www.nice.org.uk/guidance/ng51/resources/sepsis-recognition-diagnosis-and-early-management-pdf-1837508256709 (accessed 5 May 2022).

National Institute for Health and Care Excellence (NICE) (2017a) *Fractures (Complex): Assessment and Management*. Available at: www.nice.org.uk/guidance/ng37/chapter/Recommendations (accessed 15 February 2022).

National Institute for Health and Care Excellence (NICE) (2017b) *Intravenous Fluid Therapy in Adults in Hospital: Clinical Guideline [CG174]*. Available at: www.nice.org.uk/Guidance/CG174 (accessed 15 September 2022).

National Institute for Health and Care Excellence (NICE) (2017c) *Sepsis: Risk Stratification Tools*. Available at: www.nice.org.uk/guidance/ng51/resources/algorithms-and-risk-stratification-tables-compiled-version-2551488301 (accessed 1 November 2022).

National Institute for Health and Care Excellence (NICE) (2017d) *Sepsis*. Available at: www.nice.org.uk/guidance/qs161/resources/sepsis-pdf-75545595402181?msclkid=e8f8b640cf8111ecb5aa07b2488fe8c2 (accessed 5 May 2022).

References

National Institute for Health and Care Excellence (NICE) (2019a) *Stroke and Transient Ischaemic Attack in over 16s: Diagnosis and Initial Management.* Available at: www.nice.org.uk/guidance/ng128/chapter/Recommendations (accessed 28 November 2021).

National Institute for Health and Care Excellence (NICE) (2019b) *Acute Kidney Injury: Prevention, Detection and Management. NICE Guideline [NG148]* Available at: https://www.nice.org.uk/guidance/ng148/chapter/Recommendations (accessed 19 October 2022).

National Institute for Health & Care Excellence (NICE) (2020a) *Acute Coronary Syndromes.* Available at: www.nice.org.uk/guidance/ng185/resources/acute-coronary-syndromes-pdf-66142023361477 (accessed 6 December 2021).

National Institute for Health and Care Excellence (NICE) (2020b) *Sepsis: Recognition, Diagnosis and Early Treatment.* Available at: https://cks.nice.org.uk/topics/sepsis/references/ (accessed 16 September 2022).

National Institute for Health and Care Excellence (NICE) (2020c) *Stroke and TIA: Supporting Evidence.* Available at: https://cks.nice.org.uk/topics/stroke-tia/supporting-evidence/ (accessed 28 November 2021).

National Institute for Health and Care Excellence (NICE) (2021) *What Is the Prevalence of Asthma?* Available at: https://cks.nice.org.uk/topics/asthma/background-information/prevalence/ (accessed 10 November 2021).

Nursing and Midwifery Council (NMC) (2018a) *Standards of Proficiency for Nursing Associates.* London: NMC. Available at: www.nmc.org.uk/globalassets/sitedocuments/education-standards/nursing-associates-proficiency-standards.pdf (accessed 16 December 2021).

Nursing and Midwifery Council (NMC) (2018b) *Standards for Pre-registration Nursing Associate Programmes.* London: NMC. Available at: www.nmc.org.uk/globalassets/sitedocuments/standards-of-proficiency/standards-for-pre-registration-nursing-associate-programmes/nursing-associates-programme-standards.pdf (accessed 15 September 2022).

Nursing and Midwifery Council (NMC) (2018c) *Standards for Student Supervision and Assessment.* London: NMC. Available at: student-supervision-assessment.pdf (www.nmc.org.uk) (accessed 15 September 2022).

Nursing and Midwifery Council (NMC) (2018d) *The Code: Professional Standards of Practice and Behaviour for Nurses, Midwives and Nursing Associates.* London: NMC. Available at www.nmc.org.uk (accessed 15 September 2022).

Nursing and Midwifery Council (NMC) (2018e) *Future Nurse: Standards of Proficiency for Registered Nurses.* London: NMC. Available at: future-nurse-proficiencies.pdf (nmc.org.uk) (accessed 15 September 2022).

Nursing and Midwifery Council (NMC) (2019) *Revalidation: How to Revalidate with the NMC.* London: NMC. Available at: www.nmc.org.uk (accessed 15 September 2022).

Nursing and Midwifery Council (NMC) (2020) *Principles for Preceptorship.* London: NMC. Available at: nmc-principles-for-preceptorship-a5.pdf (accessed 15 September 2022).

Odelius, A., Traynor, M., Mehigan, S., Wasike, M. & Caldwell, C. (2017) Implementing and assessing the value of nursing preceptorship. *Nursing Management,* 23(9): 35–7.

Office for National Statistics (ONS) (2022) *Avoidable Mortality in Great Britain: 2020.* Available at: www.ons.gov.uk/peoplepopulationandcommunity/healthandsocialcare/causesofdeath/bulletins/avoidablemortalityinenglandandwales/latest (accessed 25 March 2022).

Peate, I. and Dutton, H. (2012) *Acute Nursing Care*. London: Taylor & Francis Group.

Peate, I. and Brent, D. (2021) Using the ABCDE approach for all critically unwell patients. *British Journal of Healthcare Assistances*, 15(2): 84–9.

Pan London Practice Learning Group (PLPLG) (2019) *The Pan London Practice Assessment Document: Nursing Associates*. Available at: https://plplg.uk/nursing-associates/ (accessed 19 October 2022).

Puthenpurakal, A. and Crussell, J. (2017) Stroke 1: Definition, burden, risk factors, diagnosis. *Nursing Times*, 113(11): 43–7.

Resuscitation Council UK (2016) *Decisions Relating to Cardiopulmonary Resuscitation: Guidance from the British Medical Association, the Resuscitation Council (UK), and the Royal College of Nursing*. Available at: www.resus.org.uk/sites/default/files/2020-05/20160123%20 Decisions%20Relating%20to%20CPR%20-%202016.pdf (accessed 28 March 2022).

Resuscitation Council UK (2021a) *Epidemiology of Cardiac Arrest Guidelines*. Available at: www. resus.org.uk/library/2021-resuscitation-guidelines/epidemiology-cardiac-arrest-guidelines (assessed 28 March 2022).

Resuscitation Council UK (2021b) *The ABCDE Approach*. Available at: www.resus.org.uk/ library/abcde-approach (accessed 28 March 2022).

Resuscitation Council UK (2021c) *Systems Saving Lives: Guidelines*. Available at: www.resus. org.uk/library/2021-resuscitation-guidelines/systems-saving-lives-guidelines (accessed 28 March 2022).

Resuscitation Council UK (2021d) *2021 Resuscitation Guidelines*. Available at: www.resus.org. uk/library/2021-resuscitation-guidelines (accessed 28 March 2022).

Resuscitation Council UK (2021e) *ReSPECT for healthcare professionals*. Available at: www. resus.org.uk/respect/respect-healthcare-professionals (accessed 28 March 2022).

Resuscitation Council UK (2021f) *Emergency Treatment of Anaphylaxis*. Available at: www. resus.org.uk/sites/default/files/2021-05/Emergency-Treatment-of-Anaphylaxis-May 2021_0. pdf (accessed 4 April 2022).

Roper, N., Logan, W. and Tierney, A. (2000) *The Roper-Logan-Tierney Model of Nursing*. Edinburgh: Churchill Livingstone.

Royal College of Physicians (RCP) (2015a) *Acute Kidney Injury and Intravenous Fluid Therapy*. Available at: www.rcplondon.ac.uk/guidelines-policy/acute-care-toolkit-12-acute-kidney-injury-and-intravenous-fluid-therapy (accessed 19 October 2022).

Royal College of Physicians (RCP) (2015b) *Why Asthma Still Kills: The National Review of Asthma Deaths (NRAD)*. Available at: www.rcplondon.ac.uk/projects/outputs/why-asthma-still-kills (accessed 10 November 2021).

Royal College of Physicians (RCP) (2017) *National Early Warning Score (NEWS) 2*. Available at: www.rcplondon.ac.uk/projects/outputs/national-early-warning-score-news-2 (accessed 28 March 2022).

Sagar, D. and Cho, J. (2022) *Neurogenic Shock*. Available at: www.ncbi.nlm.nih.gov/books/ NBK459361/ (accessed 4 April 2022).

Schwarzfuchs, D., Rabaev, E., Sagy, I., Zimhony-Nissim., N., Lipnitzki, I., Musa, H., Jotkowitz, A., Brandstaetter, E. and Barski, L. (2020). Clinical and epidemiological characteristics of diabetic ketoacidosis in older adults. *Journal of the American Geriatrics Society*, 68(6): 1256–61.

References

Sepsis Trust (2022) *Sepsis Screening and Care Tool.* Available at: https://sepsistrust.org/wp-content/uploads/2018/06/ED-adult-NICE-Final-1107.pdf (accessed 19 October 2022).

Sharma, M. and Rameshbabu, C.S. (2012). Collateral pathways in portal hypertension. *Journal of Clinical and Experimental Hepatology,* 2(4): 338–52.

Shepherd, A. (2011) Measuring and managing fluid balance. *Nursing Times* 107: 28. Available at: www.nursingtimes.net/clinical-archive/nutrition/measuring-and-managing-fluid-balance-15-07-2011/ (accessed 10 March 2022).

Singer, M., Deutschman, C.S., Seymour, C.W., Shankar-Hari, M., Annane, D., Bauer, M., Bellomo, R., Bernard, G.R., Chiche, J.D., Coopersmith, C.M., Hotchkiss, R.S., Levy, M.M., Marshall, J.C., Martin, G.S., Opal, S.M., Rubenfeld, G.D., van der Poll, T., Vincent, J.L. and Angus, D.C. (2016) The third international consensus definitions for sepsis and septic shock (Sepsis-3). *JAMA,* 315(8): 801–10.

Smith, A. (2016) *Oxford Handbook of Surgical Nursing.* Oxford: Oxford University Press.

Smith, D. and Bowden, T. (2017) Using the ABCDE approach to assess the deteriorating patient. *Nursing Standard,* 32(14): 51–63.

Smith, G. (2010) In-hospital cardiac arrest: Is it time for an in-hospital 'chain of prevention'? *Resuscitation,* 81(9): 209–11.

Stroke Association (2018) *Current, Future and Avoidable Costs of Stroke in the UK.* Available at: www.stroke.org.uk/sites/default/files/costs_of_stroke_in_the_uk_economic_case_interventions_that_work.pdf (accessed 28 November 2021).

Stroke Association (2020) *Stroke Statistics.* Available at: www.stroke.org.uk/what-is-stroke/stroke-statistics#UK (accessed 28 Novemer 2021).

Tait, D. and Hansen, S. (2016) The patient with acute kidney injury. In Tait, D., James, J., Williams, C. and Barton, D. (eds), *Acute and Critical Care in Adult Nursing* (2nd edn). London: Sage Learning Matters.

Tait, D., James, J., Williams, C. and Barton, D. (2016) *Acute and Critical Care in Adult Nursing* (2nd edn). London: Sage Learning Matters.

Tang, S.J., Hosseini-Carroll, P. and Vesa, T.S. (2019). Hemospray hemostasis in bleeding diffusely ulcerated esophagus. *VideoGIE: An Official Video Journal of the American Society for Gastrointestinal Endoscopy,* 4(3), 142–4.

Taylor, M. (2021a) Learning in and from practice. In Flaherty, C. and Taylor, M. (eds), *Practice-Based Learning for Nursing Associates.* London: Sage.

Taylor, M. (2021b) Portfolio development. In Flaherty, C. and Taylor, M. (eds), *Developing Academic Skills for Nursing Associates.* London: Sage.

Teasdale, G. (2014) Forty years on: Updating the Glasgow Coma Scale. *Nursing Times* [online], 110(42): 12–16. Available at: www.nursingtimes.net (accessed 1 November 2022).

Teasdale, G. and Jennett, B. (1974) Assessment of coma and impaired consciousness: A practical scale. *Lancet,* 2: 81–4.

Thygesen, K., Alpert, J. and Jaffe, A. et al. (2018) Fourth universal definition of myocardial infarction. *Journal of the American College of Cardiology,* 72(18): 2231–64.

Tidy, C. (2021) Femoral Fractures. Types, Symptoms and Management. https://patient.info/doctor/femoral-fractures (accessed 31 March 2022).

Tortora, G.J., and Derrickson, B.H. (2017) *Tortora's Principles of Anatomy and Physiology.* London: WILEY.

Trauma & Audit Research Network (2022) *Welcome.* Available at: www.tarn.ac.uk (accessed 16 September 2022).

Tripathi, D., Stanley, A.J., Hayes, P.C., Patch, D., Millson, C., Mehrzad, H., Austin, A., Ferguson, J.W., Olliff, S.P., Hudson, M., Christie, J.M. and Clinical Services and Standards Committee of the British Society of Gastroenterology (2015). U.K. guidelines on the management of variceal haemorrhage in cirrhotic patients. *Gut,* 64(11): 1680–704.

UK Sepsis Trust (2019) *Sepsis Screening Tool – Sepsis Six.* Available at: https://sepsistrust.org/professional-resources/clinical-tools/?msclkid=7907d578cf9e11eca8af0032f3eaddc9 (accessed 5 May 2022).

UK Sepsis Trust (2020) *The Sepsis Manual* (5th edn). *Responsible Management of Sepsis, Severe Infection and Antimicrobial Stewardship.* Available at: https://sepsistrust.org/wp-content/uploads/2020/01/5th-Edition-manual-080120.pdf (accessed 4 April 2022).

United Kingdom Health Security Agency (2015) *Act FAST Animation – Every Minute Counts.* Available at: www.youtube.com/watch?v=vc9OF64H4sE (accessed 16 December 2021).

Waterlow, J. (2005) *Waterlow Risk Assessment Score Card.* Available at: www.judy-waterlow.co.uk/the-waterlow-score-card.htm (accessed 23 November 2021).

Waugh, A. and Grant, A. (2018) *Ross and Wilson Anatomy and Physiology in Health and Illness* (14th edn). Edinburgh: Elsevier.

Weiser, T.G. and Haynes, A.B. (2018). Ten Years of the Surgical Safety Checklist. *British Journal of Surgery,* 105(8): 927–9.

Wentowski, C., Ingles, P.A. and Nielsen, N. (2021) Sepsis 2021: a review. *Anaesthesia and Intensive Care Medicine,* 22(11): 678–84.

Wettstein, A. (2020). *Investigating Teachers' Psychological and Physiological Stress.* Research OUTREACH. Available at: https://researchoutreach.org/articles/investigating-teachers-psychological-and-physiological-stress/ (accessed 20 September 2022).

Woodrow, P. (2015) *Nursing Acutely Ill Adults.* London: Taylor & Francis Group.

World Health Organization (WHO) (2016) *Human Factors: Technical Series on Safer Primary Care.* Available at: https://apps.who.int/iris/bitstream/handle/10665/252273/9789241511612-eng.pdf;sequence=1?msclkid=1339badbcfa011ec9268dad3e7016aa0 (accessed 5 May 2022).

World Health Organization (WHO) (2018) *New Checklist to Help Make Surgery Safer.* Available at: www.who.int/news/item/24-06-2008-new-checklist-to-help-make-surgery-safer (accessed 15 November 2021).

World Health Organization (WHO) (2020) *Definition of a Stroke.* Available at: www.publichealth.com.ng/world-health-organization-who-definition-of-stroke/?nowprocket=1 (accessed 28 November 2021).

Zyck, S. and Gould, G. (2021) *Cavernous Venous Malformation.* Available at: www.ncbi.nlm.nih.gov/books/NBK526009/ (accessed 16 December 2021).

Index

Locators in **bold** refer to tables and those in *italics* to figures.